# Patient Management
# Problems for the MRCPsych

# Note

This book has been written by a practising psychiatrist. All cases described in this book have been invented, and no reference to any person, in particular any former patient of the author, may be inferred.

Every effort has been taken to ensure that answers given to the clinical situations described meet with good clinical practice and the current psychiatric literature at the time of going to press, but neither the author nor the publisher can accept any liability for actions taken by the readers of this book.

Readers are also cautioned that often psychiatric practice is affected by the law, and cases described here reflect this reality. Answers to matters where the law is involved should be read in the knowledge that the author does not claim to be legally qualified, and in the event of any uncertainty, proper legal advice should be sought.

# Patient Management Problems for the MRCPsych

*Robert M Cohen, MA MBBS MRCPsych*

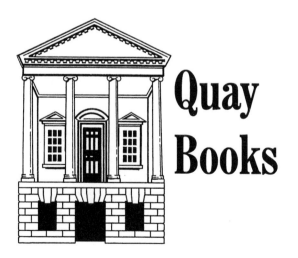

Quay Books

Quay Books Division of Mark Allen Publishing Limited
Jesse's Farm, Snow Hill, Dinton
Salisbury, Wiltshire, SP3 5HN

British Library Cataloguing-in-Publication Data
A catalogue record is available for this book

© Mark Allen Publishing Limited, 1995
ISBN 1 85642 133 3

Printed in the UK by Butler & Tanner Ltd.,
Frome and London

# Acknowledgements

This book started life as a series of individual pieces intended to help psychiatric registrars in their preparation for the MRCPsych examination. It has been published with the help of an educational grant from Lundbeck Limited, but this statement does not do justice to the support, advice and encouragement constantly offered by Dr Michael Timothy in the development of this project. He has guided the practical task of publication of the book, but responsibility for its content, including any errors that remain, is entirely mine.

All authors have to dip extensively into their private time, and in this I would like to thank my wife Liz and my son Tony for their forbearance.

# Introduction

In contrast to how it might feel to candidates, the royal colleges go some way to trying to make the membership examination represent the realities of clinical life, rather than an examination of the ability to remember exotic and unusual facts so that the specialist can make rare diagnoses. Nowhere is this more apparent than in the patient management problem section of the Part II Examination for the Membership of the Royal College of Psychiatrists (MRCPsych). With factual knowledge having been tested in other sections of the examination (multiple choice questions, short answer questions, essay paper) and examination of the patient tested in the stylised format of the long case, the patient management problem section asks whether the candidate is capable of acting as a psychiatrist in real-life clinical practice.

There is no textbook that can prepare the candidate for this part of the examination. Although the college examination supervisors check to ensure a similar standard, examiners (who are, after all, practicing psychiatrists) are asked to provide cases from their own clinical experience. Thus, the choice and type of case will vary in accordance with the different clinical encounters of individual examiners.

The result of this is that situations will be described to candidates that may have no standard answer. It may be because the diagnosis may be unclear at initial presentation, or the presentation unusual. Or it may cover the problem of handling situations where treatment is of limited efficacy or the literature is limited (for example, what to do when a patient is ill with a chronic disorder such as schizophrenia, but neuroleptics seem to be only partially effective). The case may describe a situation that a practicing clinician may encounter frequently but which is more part of the process than the disorder, and so have been afforded restricted attention in textbooks, such as how to talk to relatives of the chronically mentally ill, how to provide a useful liaison encounter on a general medical ward and how to behave as an expert psychiatric witness in court. In such cases, there may be no correct answer, but what the candidate is required to show is that he/she will approach the problem intelligently and, drawing on his/her clinical experience along with what information the literature does give, offer some sensible suggestion about how to proceed. It does not have to be the same answer as that provided by the examiner when faced with the problem in real — often different practitioners will do slightly different things when faced with similar clinical situations — but it has to be reasonable and as safe as possible.

Thus, the best preparation for this part of the examination is to get as much clinical experience as possible in the 3.5 to 4 years from becoming a trainee psychiatrist to sitting the MRCPsych examination, to spend as much time reflecting on what you see, and to take advantage of discussion with senior colleagues (especially the consultant psychiatrist in supervision sessions) and clinical colleagues from other disciplines closely related to psychiatry.

However, there is also a need to prepare for the actual examination as far as possible, and this book attempts to assist the candidate towards this. It contains 30 case `vignettes' drawn in the main from general adult psychiatry, presented in a format that allows for self-testing in conditions that mimic the examination. In the current format of this part of the examination, the candidate will meet two examiners who will each provide two vignettes over a 30-minute period, i.e. allowing 7.5 minutes per vignette. A clinical problem will be described and the candidate is required to make suggestions about how he/she would proceed. Because of the limited time available, answers can be brief and in some respects generalised (e.g. one might mention antidepressant medication as one of several treatment options, without needing to specify which antidepressant and why, unless that is the focus of the problem): discussion of any point will have to be limited.

In this book, questions are presented in a format that can be read aloud and a suggested set of answers is provided on the next page. It can, therefore, be used for private study or for study in a group where one person can act as `examiner', and then other members of the group can offer suggestions as to how they would proceed. Answers generated may differ somewhat in both format and content from what is suggested by the author, but this will not necessarily invalidate either. It should be noted that in many of the vignettes there are more parts than can be easily dealt with in 7.5 minutes, and those using the vignettes as mock examinations should try to limit them accordingly; the longer versions allow more material to be brought into the book.

The list for further reading at the end of each vignette is not intended to be exhaustive: it may indicate the source of some particular point in the answer given; it may indicate an earlier paper that was germinal in the development of that branch of psychiatry; or it may contain more general discussion of the topic in the vignette and related matters. Suggestions, comments and criticisms (politely phrased, please!) about the vignettes, the answers or the reading lists will be welcomed by the author.

Psychiatry is a most fascinating and intellectually stimulating branch of medicine, allowing for consideration of how the mind works in health and disease, both alone and in relation to the body, along with a host of social, legal, moral, ethical and philosophical issues. The stimulants to this quest are to be found in the clinical examinations carried out daily. Although the prime focus of this book will be, for many readers, a practical aid to the patient management problem section of the MRCPsych examination, I hope that it will also prove an enjoyable journey.

*Robert Cohen, January 1995*

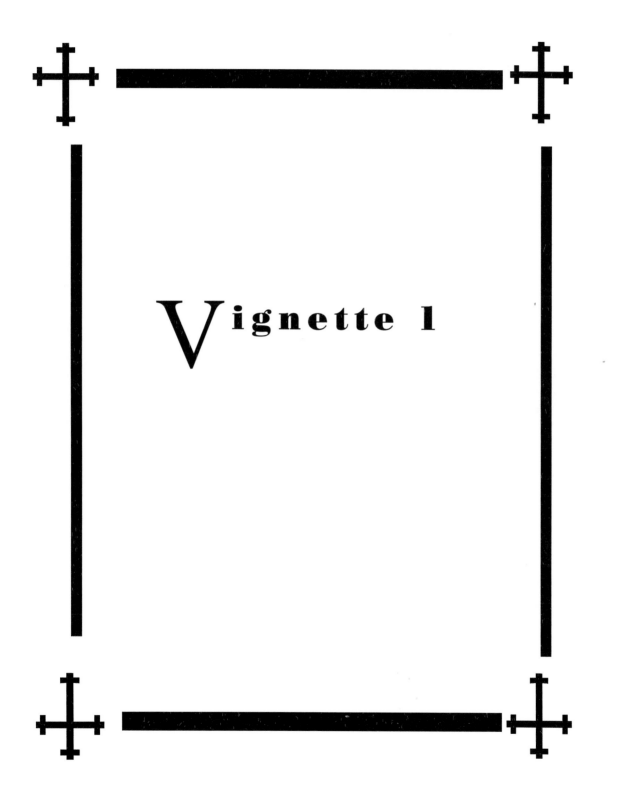

Vignette 1

# Vignette 1

*You are called by the sister of the acute psychiatric admission ward who tells you that a man in his late 20s who was admitted earlier in the afternoon with an exacerbation of known paranoid schizophrenia has smashed two windows on the ward in response to voices telling him that he is going to be murdered by the IRA if he stays on the ward. What are the principles of management of the acute violent situation?*

You are called by the sister of the acute psychiatric admission ward who tells you that a man in his late 20s who was admitted earlier in the afternoon with an exacerbation of known paranoid schizophrenia has smashed two windows on the ward in response to voices telling him that he is going to be murdered by the IRA if he stays on the ward. What are the principles of management of the acute violent situation?

- Containment of the situation

- Reduction in the acute distress of the patient, primarily with medication

- Reassurance to other patients and staff after the event

*How is this achieved?*

## How is this achieved?

1. Containment of the situation:

   - Ensure adequate numbers of staff (police if necessary)
   - Establish who is in charge (ward manager, junior doctor) and act confidently
   - Remove people who are not involved (other patients, visitors) from the immediate area
   - Allow a distressed and volatile patient plenty of room: do not pressurise him
   - Restrain the patient
   - Consider nursing in a seclusion room, removing objects that can be used as weapons.

2. Reduction in the acute distress of the patient, primarily with medication:

   - Reassure the patient that he is safe and that his hallucinations will not happen. Do not argue with him
   - Administer intramuscular neuroleptic medication (haloperidol, chlorpromazine (inadvisable) or acuphase [zuclopenthixol acetate])
   - Administer intravenous benzodiazepine.

3. Reassurance to other patients and staff after the event:

   - Informal discussion with staff members over a cup of tea
   - Informal counseling by nursing staff of distressed patients
   - Discussion in the ward meeting.

*What should you do after the immediate event?*

## What should you do after the immediate event?

- Ensure that you are adequately prepared for the management of future incidents

- Ensure that you know how to use neuroleptic medication in the acute situation.

# Further reading

Anonymous (1991) Management of behavioural emergencies. *Drug Ther Bull* **29**: 62–4

Breakwell GM (1989) *Facing Physical Violence*. British Psychological Society/Routledge, Leicester/London

Carmel H, Hunter M (1989) Staff injuries from inpatient violence. *Hosp Community Psychiatry* **40**: 41–6

Fisher WA (1994) Restraint and seclusion: a review of the literature. *Am J Psychiatry* **151**: 1584–91

Fottrell E (1980) A study of violent behaviour among patients in psychiatric hospitals. *Br J Psychiatry* **136**: 216–21

Fottrell E (1981) Violent behaviour by psychiatric patients. *Br J Hosp Med* **25**(1): 28–38

Haller RM, Deluty RH (1988) Assaults on staff by psychiatric inpatients: a critical review. *Br J Psychiatry* **152**: 174–9

Health and Safety Commission (1988) *Violence to Staff in the Health Services*. HMSO, London

Howells K, Hollin C R eds. (1989) *Clinical Approaches to Violence*. John Wiley, Chichester (especially chapters 12 & 13)

Hyman SE (1988) *Manual of Psychiatric Emergencies*. Little, Brown and Co. Boston

James DV, Fineberg NA, Shah AK, Priest RG (1990) An increase in violence on an acute psychiatric ward. A study of associated factors. *Br J Psychiatry* **156**: 846–52

McGrath G, Bowker M (1987) *Common Psychiatric Emergencies*. Wright, Bristol

Pfeffer JM (1981) Management of the acutely disturbed patient on the general ward. *Br J Hosp Med* **26**(1): 73–8

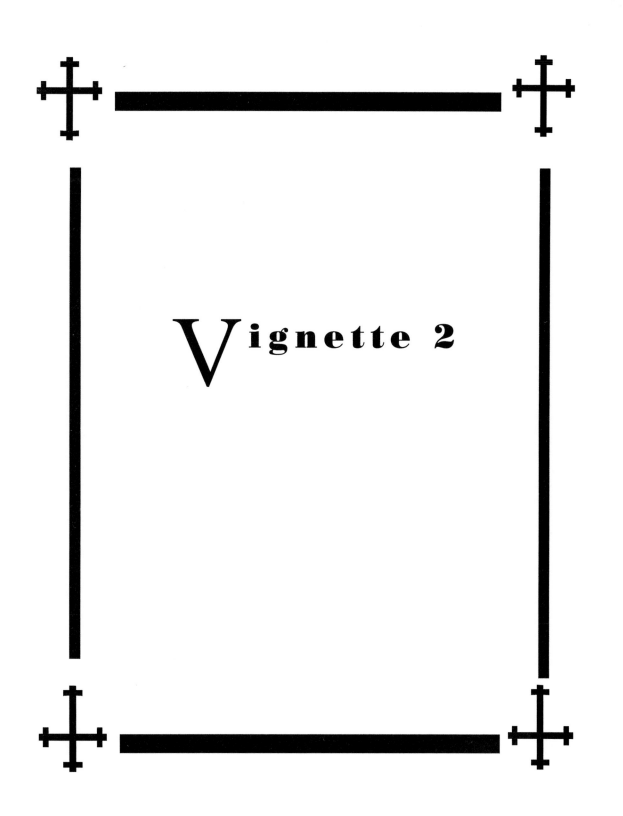

Vignette 2

# Vignette 2

*A 27-year-old man has been an inpatient on the acute psychiatric admission ward for the last 8 weeks following a second episode of illness characterised by third-person auditory hallucinations, somatic hallucinations, thought broadcasting and paranoid delusions. He has responded well to the oral neuroleptic drug on which he was started. How do you start the formal process of planning his aftercare?*

*What is the name of the Government initiative for planning aftercare?*

A 27-year-old man has been an inpatient on the acute psychiatric admission ward for the last 8 weeks following a second episode of illness characterised by third-person auditory hallucinations, somatic hallucinations, thought broadcasting and paranoid delusions. He has responded well to the oral neuroleptic drug on which he was started. How do you start the formal process of planning his aftercare?

● Call a discharge planning meeting (or section 117 meeting if the patient has been admitted under section 3). This may be done at the time of a ward round.

**What is the name of the Government initiative for planning aftercare?**

● The Care Programme Approach.

*Who might be involved in the aftercare of the patient and thus needed at any clinical planning meeting?*

*What are the formal guidelines for psychiatrists planning aftercare?*

## Who might be involved in the aftercare of the patient and thus needed at any clinical planning meeting?

- The patient

- The consultant psychiatrist/junior psychiatric staff

- The patient's general practitioner

- The community psychiatric nurse

- A social worker

- A key worker

- A worker from the patient's residential home/day placement/work

- Relatives or advocates of the patient.

## What are the formal guidelines for psychiatrists planning aftercare?

- The Royal College of Psychiatrists (1991) has produced a document entitled *Good Medical Practice in the Aftercare of Potentially Violent or Vulnerable Patients Discharged from Inpatient Psychiatric Treatment* (October 1991).

*What is the role of the psychiatrist in aftercare?*

*What is the principle of medication and what options are available?*

## What is the role of the psychiatrist in aftercare?

- Arranging for regular reviews of the patient (outpatient follow-up, community psychiatric nurse, informal liaison with key worker, social worker and general practitioner)

- Advice about medication

- Advice about family therapy with respect to dealing with high expressed emotion

- Advice about accommodation requirements (hospital hostel, residential hostel, group homes, landlady schemes, living with relatives, independent living)

- Advice about fitness for work or other occupational resource

- Ensuring his/her part of a rapid response mechanism should the patient exhibit symptoms and/or signs of relapse.

## What are the principles and the options of medication?

- Neuroleptic medication in maintenance doses, either orally or by regular depot injection.

*What are the advantages and disadvantages of oral versus depot medication?*

# What are the advantages and disadvantages of oral versus depot medication?

1.  Oral medication:

| Advantages | Disadvantages |
|---|---|
| • Short duration<br>• Flexibility | • Poor compliance<br>• Misuse<br>• Taken daily (several times) |

2.  Depot medication:

| Advantages | Disadvantages |
|---|---|
| • Compliance<br>• Improved bioavailability<br><br>• No problem with absorption/ ↓ first-pass effect<br>• Reduces risk of abuse or overdose<br>• Amount of drug taken accurately<br>• Regular contact with community psychiatric nurse | • Delay in side-effects<br>• If patient suffers side-effects, these can take longer to wear off<br>• Needles<br><br>• Abscess formation |

> *How does one go about starting this patient on a depot neuroleptic drug?*

## How does one go about starting this patient on a depot neuroleptic drug?

- Test dose

- Increase the depot medication at regular intervals (e.g. weekly)

- Decrease oral medication and eventually stop it

- Reduce depot medication to maintenance levels

- Review the patient regularly (e.g. depot clinic).

# Further reading

Department of Health and Welsh Office (1990). *Code of Practice – Mental Health Act 1983*, HMSO, London (chapter 26 on aftercare)

Hirsch SR (1986). Clinical treatment of schizophrenia. In: Bradley PB, Hirsch SR, eds. *The Psychopharmacology and Treatment of Schizophrenia*. Oxford University Press, Oxford

Leff J, Vaughn C (1981). The role of maintenance therapy and relatives expressed emotion in relapse of schizophrenia. A two-year follow-up. *Br J Psychiatry*, **139**: 102–4

The Royal College of Psychiatrists (1991) *Good Medical Practice in the Aftercare of Potentially Violent or Vulnerable Patients Discharged from Inpatient Psychiatric Treatment*. Royal College of Psychiatrists, London

The Royal College of Psychiatrists (1993) *Patient Factsheet. Depot Antipsychotic Medication: What You Should Know*. Royal College of Psychiatrists, London

Vaugn C, Leff J (1976) The influence of family and social factors on the course of psychiatric illness. *Br J Psychiatry*, **129**: 125–37

Wistedt B, Gerlach J, eds, (1990) *Depot Antipsychotics in Chronic Schizophrenia*. Elsevier, Amsterdam

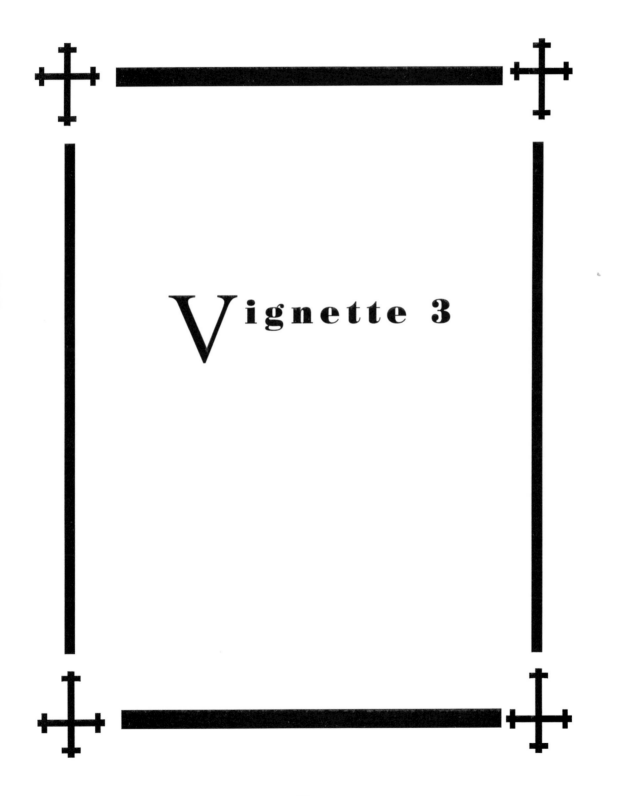

Vignette 3

# Vignette 3

*You are asked to review a 24-year-old man in a ward round. He has been an inpatient for 4 weeks, having been admitted with the belief that he is being pursued by the IRA. He says that he knows this because he can hear things like `He's not going to get away', being broadcast over the airwaves. He has been treated while an inpatient with haloperidol, but there has been no change in his mental state. What things do you look at and what do you do?*

You are asked to review a 24-year-old man in a ward round. He has been an inpatient for 4 weeks, having been admitted with the belief that he is being pursued by the IRA because he can hear things like 'He's not going to get away', being broadcast over the airwaves. He has been treated while an inpatient with haloperidol, but there has been no change in his mental state. What things do you look at and what do you do?

- Check that the neuroleptic drug has been prescribed in the patient's pharmacy card

- Check the dose

- Check the length of time the patient has been on this dose

- Review the psychiatric notes for any previous episodes, what medication and which dose the patient required and how long the patient needed before responding

- Check whether the patient has a medical condition that might aggravate the mental state by itself or through its treatment (e.g. Cushing's syndrome or treatment with corticosteroids)

- Check whether the patient has been taking the tablets by asking the nurses whether the patient has been refusing medication, whether medication has not been available from the pharmacy, if they have any reason to suspect that the patient is throwing his tablets away (hiding them in his cheek, throwing themdown the toilet, giving them to other patients) or whether the patient has missed doses because of not being on the ward at times for medication (not getting back from leave on time, periods of absconding)

- Check if the patient might be taking any illicit/hallucinogenic substance (cannabis, cocaine, amphetamines) that might prevent recovery

- Check whether the pharmacy has recently changed its supplier of haloperidol

- Ensure that the patient receives the drug in a sufficient dose for a sufficient length of time

- Consider changing the formulation (e.g. tablet to syrup, depot)

- Consider using a different neuroleptic drug

- Do not sanction periods of leave

- Take urine drug screens after periods of absence from the ward.

*Several months later, the patient is still on the ward and has not experienced any remission from his symptoms despite taking successively three different conventional neuroleptic drugs in adequate doses, and with no confounding factors as suggested earlier. How do you manage the patient now and what other treatment options are available to you?*

**Several months later, the patient is still on the ward and has not experienced any remission from his symptoms despite taking successively three different conventional neuroleptic drugs in adequate doses, and with no confounding factors as suggested earlier. How do you manage the patient now and what other treatment options are available to you?**

1.    Review the diagnosis:

    ●   Review the patient's case notes
    ●   Consider taking an electroencephalogram/computed tomography (EEG/CT) scan if not already done.

2.    Consider drug treatment options:

    ●   Depot neuroleptic drug
    ●   Augmentative therapy — (neuroleptic + benzodiazepine/lithium/ propranolol)
    ●   Second line drug — (clozapine).

3.    Consider other therapies:

    ●   Walkman audiocassette, ear plugs, subvocal counting/singing to oneself for auditory hallucinations if they continue to be distressing (although be aware that chronic patients may learn to live with their voices)
    ●   Review stressors that might prevent remission.

# Further reading

Angrist B, Schulz SC, eds, (1990) *The Neuroleptic Non-Responsive Patient.* American Psychiatric Press, Washington, DC

*British Journal of Psychiatry* (1992. Clozapine — the atypical antipsychotic, *Br J Psychiatry* **160**: Supp.17

Connell PH (1958) *Amphetamine psychosis, Maudsley Monograph No 5.* Chapman & Hall, London

Davison K, Bagley CR (1969) Schizophrenia-like psychoses associated with organic disorders of the central nervous system: a review of the literature. In: Herrington RN, ed. *Current Problems in Neuropsychiatry British Journal of Psychiatry Special Publication No 4.* Headley Bros, Ashford

Donaldson SR, Gelenberg AJ, Baldessarini RJ (1983) The pharmacologic treatment of schizophrenia: a progress report. *Schizophrenia Bull* **9**: 504–27

Hale A (1993). Will the new antipsychotics improve the treatment of schizophrenia? *Br Med J* 307: 749–50

Hall RCW, Popkin MK, Stickney SK, Gardner ER (1979) Presentation of the steroid psychoses. *J Nerv Ment Dis* 167: 229–36

Huckle PL, Palia SS (1993) Managing resistant schizophrenia, *Br J Hosp Med* **50**: 467--71

McGuire P, Fahy T (1991) Chronic paranoid psychosis after misuse of MDMA (`ecstasy'). *Br Med J* **302**: 697

Nelson HE, Thrasher S, Barnes TRE (1991) Practical ways of alleviating auditory hallucinations *Br Med J* 302: 327

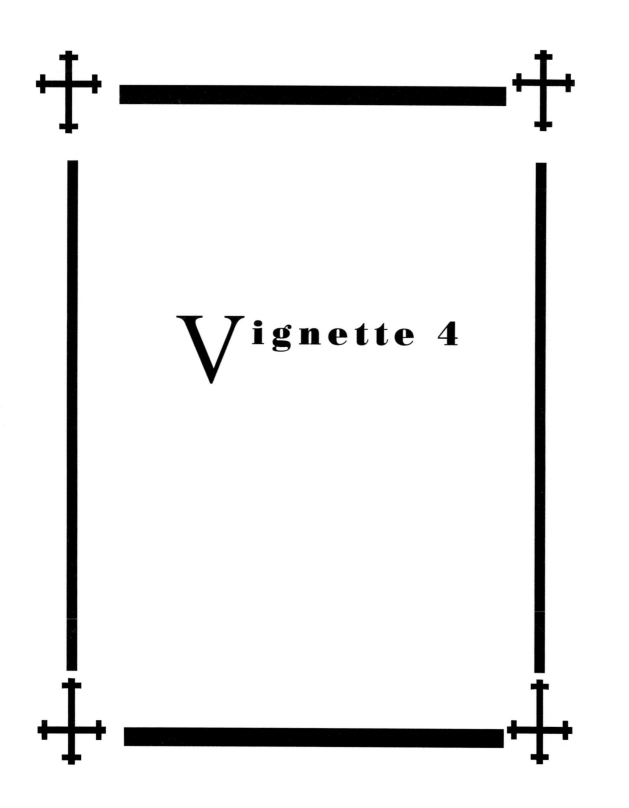

Vignette 4

# Vignette 4

A 36-year-old man has been in hospital for 3 weeks following his second hypomanic episode in a year. His mental state has settled satisfactorily on haloperidol. He has agreed to take lithium prophylactically. How do you prepare him for lithium therapy and how do you initiate and monitor treatment?

**A 36-year-old man has been in hospital for 3 weeks following his second hypomanic episode in a year. His mental state has settled satisfactorily on haloperidol. He has agreed to take lithium prophylactically. How do you prepare him for lithium therapy and how do you initiate and monitor treatment?**

1.  Preparation for lithium therapy:

    - Send blood sample to the laboratory to test for urea and electrolyte levels, and thyroid function
    - Give creatinine clearance tests.

2.  Treatment initiation:

    - Start at a low dose (e.g. 400 mg at night)
    - After a few days, check his lithium level at 11–13 hours after the last dose
    - If it is not in the therapeutic range (usually 0.4–1.0 mmol/litre but there will be some variation between laboratories), raise the dose by, for example 200 mg at night
    - After a few days, again check his lithium level at 11–13 hours after the last dose
    - Repeat this process of gradually increasing the dose and checking the level until a dose is reached which yields a therapeutic plasma level
    - Recheck the plasma level at weekly intervals for 3 weeks
    - Recheck the plasma level at monthly intervals for 3 months.

3.  Treatment maintenance:

    - Check the plasma lithium level every 3 months
    - Check urea and electrolyte levels, administer serum creatinine and thyroid function tests every 6 months
    - Some clinicians perform a yearly creatinine clearance test.

*What are the side-effects of lithium at therapeutic levels and what are the clinical indications of lithium toxicity?*

# What are the side-effects of lithium at therapeutic levels and what are the clinical indications of lithium toxicity?

1.   Side-effects of lithium at therapeutic levels:

- Weight gain
- Polyuria/polydipsia
- Inhibition of antidiuretic hormone, renal impairment
- Fine tremor
- Lithium-induced hypothyroidism
- Metallic taste in mouth
- Toxic interaction with haloperidol.

2.   Indication of lithium toxicity:

- Coarse tremor
- Ataxia, slurring of speech
- Lowered level of consciousness, coma.

*What options are available as second-line treatment if lithium therapy is unsuccessful in maintaining the patient?*

## What options are available as second-line treatment if lithium therapy is unsuccessful in maintaining the patient?

- Addition or substitution of carbamazepine

- Use of sodium valproate

- Addition or substitution of chronic neuroleptic drugs in oral or depot form (especially flupenthixol)

- Buproprion

- L-thyroxine.

# Further reading

Aronson JK, Reynolds DJM (1992) ABC of monitoring drug therapy: lithium. *Br Med J* **305**: 1273–6

Baastrup PC, Poula JC, Schou M, Thomsen K, Amdisen A (1970) Prophylactic lithium: double-blind discontinuation in manic-depressive and recurrent depressive disorders. *Lancet* **ii**: 326–30

Elphick M (1989). Clinical issues in the use of carbamazepine in psychiatry: a review. *Psychol Med* **19**: 591–604

Johnson FN, ed. (1987) *Depression and Mania - Modern Lithium Therapy*. IRL Press, Oxford

Makanjuola ROA (1985) Recurrent unipolar manic disorder in the Yoruba Nigerian: further evidence. *Br J Psychiatry* **147**: 434–7

Schou M (1986) Lithium therapy: a refresher course. *Br J Psychiatry* **149**: 541–7

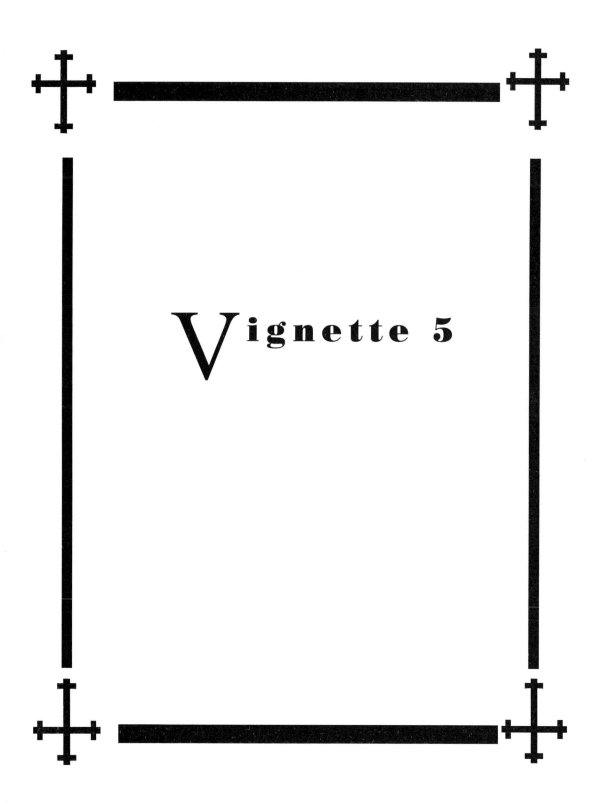

Vignette 5

# Vignette 5

*A 29-year-old clerical officer comes to the casualty department saying that for the last 6 weeks he has been finding it increasingly hard to keep up with the growing demands at work, where `company restructuring' has reduced the number of staff in his department and where he says that colleagues from other departments, themselves under pressure, are writing their request forms to him in increasingly illegible handwriting. He says that one week ago he had influenza, with aches and pains in his bones, headaches and a blocked-up nose; he feels miserable, sniffly, finds it hard to concentrate and cannot even be bothered to watch the television. The only other possibly medically relevant detail in his history is that 3 years previously, he was admitted to a mental hospital for 4 weeks, when he was treated with chlorpromazine, but there was no follow-up after discharge. On examination, he has a pyrexia of 37.3°C, but no other signs are apparent. What is the differential diagnosis?*

A 29-year-old clerical officer comes to the casualty department saying that for the last 6 weeks he has been finding it increasingly hard to keep up with the growing demands at work, where 'company restructuring' has reduced the number of staff in his department and where he says that colleagues from other departments, themselves under pressure, are writing their request forms to him in increasingly illegible handwriting. He says that one week ago he had influenza, with aches and pains in his bones, headaches and a blocked-up nose; he feels miserable, sniffly, finds it hard to concentrate and cannot even be bothered to watch the television. The only other possibly medically relevant detail in his history is that 3 years previously, he was admitted to a mental hospital for 4 weeks, when he was treated with chlorpromazine, but there was no follow-up after discharge. On examination, he has a pyrexia of 37.3°C, but no other signs are apparent. What is the differential diagnosis?

- Influenza

- Overwork

- 'Postviral fatigue'

- Neurotic depression.

*Having discharged him home with a diagnosis of influenza, he returns the next night to the casualty department. As you saw him the previous night, the casualty officer asks you to see him again. He is unable to give a history because, although he is alert, he is overactive, restless, agitated and tearful, and he believes that space invaders are chasing him, saying "This brain is why it is all happening. You do understand don't you?" while drawing a picture of a brain on a piece of paper and writing on the paper "The brain. 666. Buy more Weetabix and milk". What do you do now and what diagnoses do you consider?*

Having discharged him home with a diagnosis of influenza, he returns the next night to the casualty department. As you saw him the previous night, the casualty officer asks you to see him again. He is unable to give a history because, although he is alert, he is overactive, restless, agitated and tearful, and he believes that space invaders are chasing him, saying "This brain is why it is all happening. You do understand don't you?" while drawing a picture of a brain on a piece of paper and writing on the paper "The brain. 666. Buy more Weetabix and milk". What do you do now and what diagnoses do you consider?

1.  Examine the patient carefully, for signs of a physical illness:.

    ● If there are signs of acute physical illness (pyrexia, tachycardia, lowered level of consciousness, neck stiffness), the differential diagnosis would include an acute confusional state (due to infection, perhaps with signs of septicaemia), meningitis or encephalitis, and the patient should be referred to a physician for medical admission and management. You should offer to review the patient when the medical emergency has been treated if psychiatric symptoms and signs are still present.

2.  If nothing can be found on physical examination, the diagnosis is probably a psychiatric one and at this stage should include:

    ● Schizophrenia
    ● Schizoaffective psychosis
    ● Psychotic depression
    ● Delirium tremens.

*Define schizoaffective disorder*

## Define schizoaffective disorder.

This is an episodic disorder in which both affective and schizophrenic symptoms are prominent within the same episode of illness, preferably simultaneously, but at least within a few days of each other (ICD–10, F25: World Health Organization, 1992))

A disturbance during which, at some time, there is either a major depressive or a manic syndrome concurrent with symptoms that meet the 'A criterion' of schizophrenia, with a period of disturbance without mood symptoms for 2 weeks, that Schizophrenia has been ruled out and an organic factor has not initiated and maintained the disturbance (DSM–IV, 295.70: American Psychiatric Association, 1994)

- Typical age of onset in early adulthood

- Tendency towards a chronic course, with prognosis better than that for schizophrenia but worse than that for mood disorder

- Family studies indicate increased risk of schizophrenia in first-degree relatives and, perhaps, an increased risk of mood disorder in relatives.

*What are the principles of management of schizoaffective disorder?*

# What are the principles of management of schizoaffective disorder?

1.     Pharmacological treatment tends to be symptomatic:

- Neuroleptic drugs, oral or depot, for schizophrenic symptoms
- Lithium, antidepressant drugs for affective symptoms.

2.     Avoid psychotomimetics

3.     General treatment of chronic mental illness

- Attention to social factors — accommodation, occupation, finances and social support.

# Further reading

American Psychiatric Association (1994) *Diagnostic and Statistical Manual of Mental Disorders*. 4th edn. American Psychiatric Association, Washington DC

Brockington I, Leff J (1979). Schizoaffective psychosis: definitions and incidence, *Psycholog Med* **9**: 91–9

Fish F (1984) Schizoaffective psychoses. In: Hamilton M, ed. *Fish's Schizophrenia.*, Wright, PSG, Bristo:l 111–5

Grossman LS (1990) Long-term course and outcome in schizoaffective disorders. *Curr Op Psychiatry* **3**: 38–42

Lowe MR, Batchelor DH (1990) Lithium and neuroleptics in the management of manic-depressive psychosis. *Human Psychopharmacol* **5**: 267–74

Procci WR (1976) Schizoaffective psychosis: fact or fiction? *Arch Gen Psychiatry* **33**: 1167–78

World Health Organization (1992) *The ICD0–10 Classification of Mental and Behavioural Disorders: Clinical Description and Diagnostic Guidelines*. World Health Organization, Geneva

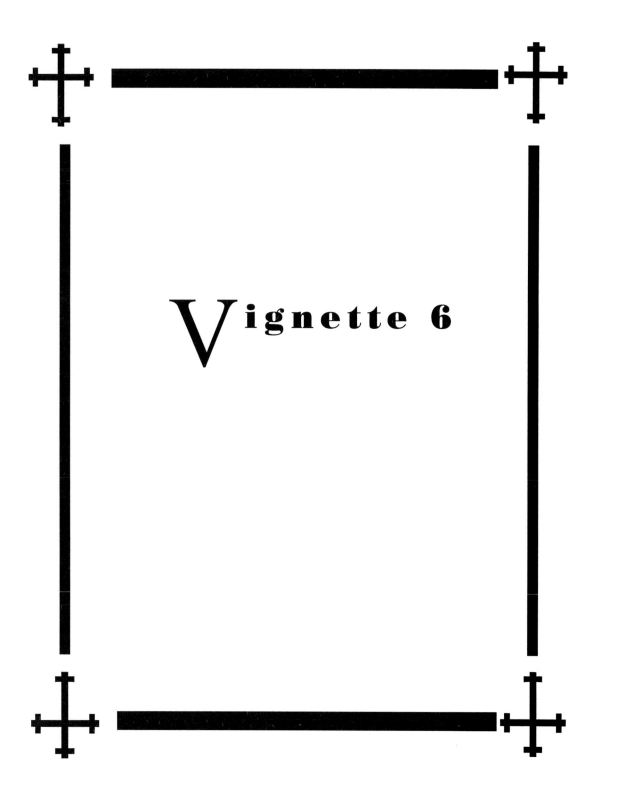

Vignette 6

# Vignette 6

*You are telephoned by a GP who says that he has been contacted by the wife of a 74-year-old man because, this morning, he threw over his bowl of cereal, and the wife is saying "I don't know what's gotten into him". She wants something to make him right and the GP is ringing to ask you what he should prescribe. How do you handle the situation?*

**You are telephoned by a GP who says that he has been contacted by the wife of a 74-year-old man because, this morning, he threw over his bowl of cereal, and the wife is saying "I don't know what's gotten into him". She wants something to make him right and the GP is ringing to ask you what he should prescribe. How do you handle the situation?**

The information you have been given is inadequate to make a diagnosis. It would, therefore, be very unwise to give any advice over the telephone at this stage. However, if you are pressured into doing so, you should record what the GP tells you in notes written during the conversation ('contemporaneous notes') and clearly document what advice you gave and your reasons.

Assuming that you have refused, at this stage, to make a diagnosis or give advice, ensure that the GP has seen the patient and excluded physical illness.

If this is the case, offer to do a domiciliary visit and discuss with the GP how urgent he thinks it is.

While on the telephone, take the opportunity to find out from the GP details of:
- Past medical and psychiatric history
- Current medical problems
- Medication that the patient is currently taking
- Allergies
- Any social history that the GP can give:

    i. Who is the main carer?

    ii. Is there any statutory support, such as a social worker or district nurse?

    iii. Are any other important relatives or friends involved; are there any underlying issues that might constitute a hidden agenda for any of the referring persons?

In this case, it may be a good idea to use a telephone call to arrange an appointment to gain some initial history from the patient's wife to assess the possibility of violence when you visit (in which case, it is unwise to visit alone).

*The GP, who from past experience you know to be a good GP, tells you that, in fact, he did visit the previous afternoon, has examined the patient physically and confirms that he cannot find any physical problem to account for what has happened. He adds that, just to be sure, he has sent off routine blood tests to your hospital's pathology laboratory. You agree to carry out a domiciliary visit. What diagnostic possibilities should you be considering as you set out?*

The GP, who from past experience you know to be a good GP, tells you that, in fact, he did visit the previous afternoon, has examined the patient physically and confirms that he cannot find any physical problem to account for what has happened. He adds that, just to be sure, he has sent off routine blood tests to your hospital's pathology laboratory. You agree to carry out a domiciliary visit. What diagnostic possibilities should you be considering as you set out?

- Marital disharmony

- Depressive illness

- Cognitive impairment due to a dementing process.

*Give 10 different types of dementia*

## Give 10 different types of dementia.

- Alzheimer's disease

- Multi-infarct dementia

- Alcoholic dementia

- Parkinson's disease

- Subcortical dementia — Lewy body disease

- Dementia of the frontal lobe type

- Pick's disease

- Normal pressure hydrocephalus

- Huntington's disease (chorea!!!)

- Binzwanger's disease

- Creutzfeld–Jacob disease

- Dementia due to cerebral metastases

- Dementia due to cerebral abscess

- Dementia post-head injury

- Boxer's dementia (dementia pugilistica)

- Acquired immunodeficiency syndrome dementia

- General Paresis of the Insane (GPI).

*After visiting the patient and carrying out a thorough psychiatric examination of his mental state and obtaining informant history from his wife (who is very fond of him and appropriately concerned about him), you make a clinical diagnosis that the patient is suffering from a dementing illness, with irritability and a depressive component. You telephone the GP to convey your findings and discuss the case with him. The GP, listening carefully to what you are saying, asks for advice about the principles of physical treatments in dementia. How do you answer?*

**After visiting the patient and carrying out a thorough psychiatric examination of his mental state and obtaining informant history from his wife (who is very fond of him and appropriately concerned about him), you make a clinical diagnosis that the patient is suffering from a dementing illness, with irritability and a depressive component. You telephone the GP to convey your findings and discuss the case with him. The GP, listening carefully to what you are saying, asks for advice about the principles of physical treatments in dementia. How do you answer?**

There is no pharmacological treatment of dementia at present, although research is being carried out into the efficacy of drugs that enhance cholinergic transmission in the brain.

The role of neuroleptic drugs in the treatment of agitation, irritability and sleep disturbance is mainly for their effects as tranquillisers, and there is always a need to balance their sedative effect with the risk that they (and any other drug that works as a CNS depressant, such as a benzodiazepine or a chloral derivative) might increase the confusion and make the situation worse. However, empirically it has been found that some patients benefit from a small dose of a neuroleptic drug on a regular basis, therefore making management of the patient easier. This could mean the difference between allowing a relative to continue caring for the patient at home for a little longer, and hospitalisation. For patients who benefit from the use of neuroleptic drugs in this way but who are unreliable in taking the medication (i.e. because they forget or resist each time they are given a pill), a small dose of a depot neuroleptic drug may be a useful strategy.

There is clinical research evidence that if a patient with dementia has a depressive component, he may benefit from antidepressant treatment for his mood, even if this does not enhance his cognitive performance. Note that the tricyclics have anticholinergic side-effects (including postural hypotension that may precipitate falls, bladder retention and bowel slowing that may lead to overflow incontinence, and the anticholinergic effect plus any sedative effect may interfere with cognitive function) but selective serotonin reuptake inhibitors (SSRIs) can cause a serotonergic syndrome. Thus, using antidepressant medication in this group is always a question of weighing up risks and benefits.

# Further Reading

Baldwin RC, Benbow SM, Marriott A, Tomenson B (1993) Depression in old age. A reconsideration of cerebral disease in relation to outcome. *Br J Psychiatry* **163**: 82–90

Carter J, Anderson B (1994) Molecular pathology of Alzheimer's disease. *Br J Hosp Med* **51**: 522–8

Howard R, Levy R (1993) Depot antipsychotic medication in the management of behavioural and psychotic symptoms in dementia? *Int J Ger Psychiatry* **8**: 111–3

Katzman R (1986) Alzheimer's disease (review). *N Engl J Med* **314**: 964–73

Lishman WA (1987) *Organic Psychiatry — The Psychological Consequences of Cerebral Disorder*. Blackwell Scientific, Oxford

Rossor M (1993) Alzheimer's disease, (fortnightly review). *Br Med J* **307**: 779–82

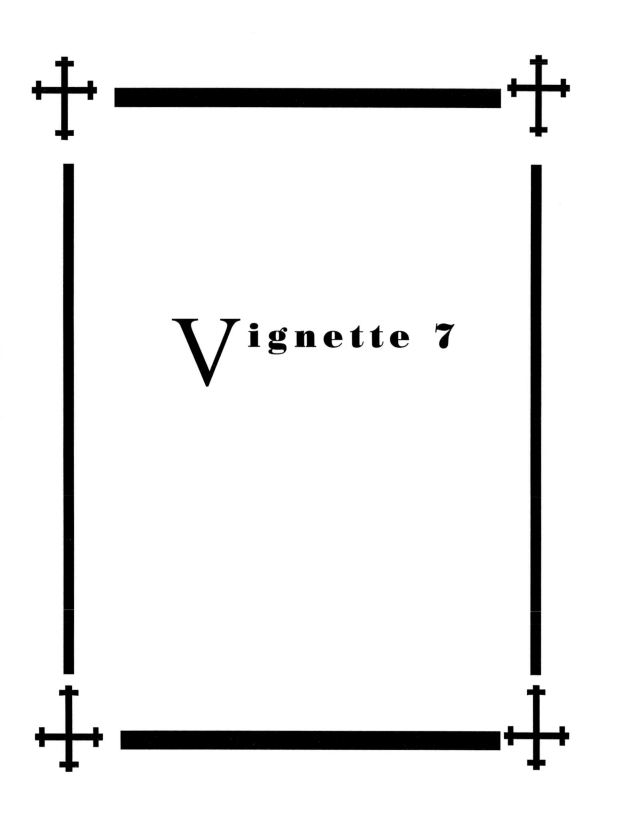

# Vignette 7

# Vignette 7

*You are called by the medical registrar to advise about a 65-year-old married man who had been admitted 2 weeks ago with a left hemiparesis which is now resolving but who is having crying spells. What possible diagnoses go through your mind as you go to the ward?*

You are called by the medical registrar to advise about a 65-year-old married man who had been admitted 2 weeks ago with a left hemiparesis which is now resolving but who is having crying spells. What possible diagnoses go through your mind as you go to the ward?

- Non-specific reaction to an episode of serious illness

- Post-stroke emotionalism

- Depressive illness (post-stroke or independent)

- Cognitive impairment (either acute confusional state or dementing process).

*How do you carry out a liaison assessment on a general medical ward?*

## How do you carry out a liaison assessment on a general medical ward?

- Introduce yourself to the nursing staff

- Take the patient's history from the referring doctor, nursing staff and patient's relatives if available

- Consult the medical notes to understand the nature of the current medical illness, the past medical history and treatment received that might be influencing the mental state or confusing the assessment of the mental state, and to gain evidence of other assessments that have been made (occupational therapy, speech therapy, physiotherapy, psychology assessments)

- Examine the patient, if possible in private (only if unavoidable examine the patient in his bed), and take a full history noting the mental state

- After completing the assessment, write a comprehensive note in the formulation format. Direct verbal communication of your findings to the nursing staff and the referring doctor assists good relations between the disciplines of psychiatry and general medicine.

*What are the clinical differences that distinguish post-stroke emotionalism from depression?*

## What are the clinical differences that distinguish post-stroke emotionalism from depression?

- Onset of emotion is sudden

- Emotional expression is uncontrollable by the patient

- The emotion is socially inappropriate in its expression

- The patient exhibits emotion while claiming that he does not feel it ("I don't know why I'm crying. I'm not unhappy")

- Episodes of emotionalism last from seconds to a few minutes, although they can occasionally last for a few hours

- It is occasionally associated with pathological laughter in the same patient.

*How would you treat post-stroke emotionalism?*

## How would you treat post-stroke emotionalism?

1.   Re-assurance

   - That the symptom is common
   - That it improves with time

2.   Drug therapy

   - Tricyclic antidepressants/SSRI
   - Levodopa
   - TRH

# Further reading

Anderson G, Vestergaard K, Riis JO (1993) Citalopram for post-stroke pathological crying. *Lancet* **343**: 816–7

Allman P (1991) Depressive disorders and emotionalism following stroke. *Int J Ger Psychiatry*, **6**: 377–83

House A (1987) Depression after stroke. *Br Med J* **i**: 76

House A (1987) Mood disorders after stroke: a review of the evidence *Int J Ger Psychiatric* **2**: 211–21

Oyebode F, Kennedy S, Davison K (1986) Psychiatric sequelae of subarachnoid haemorrhage. *Br J Hosp Med*, **36**(2): 104–8

van Gijn J (1993) Treating uncontrolled crying after stroke. *Lancet* **343**: 816–7

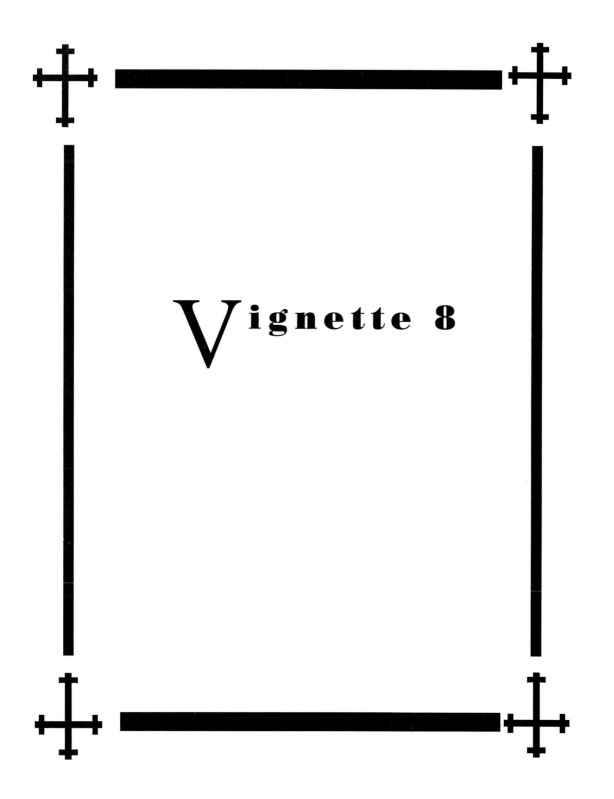

Vignette 8

# Vignette 8

*A 27-year-old woman presents to you in the routine outpatient clinic with the belief that she was receiving special signs from the newspapers telling her that she had been singled out to perform a mission to save the world, and had started hearing voices telling her how to carry out her mission. She agrees that some of what has happened to her may be a trick of her mind, but not all. She agrees with you that she might be having a nervous breakdown, but is unwilling to come into hospital. What features would make hospital admission advisable and what features would make you content to treat her as an outpatient?*

A 27-year-old woman presents to you in the routine outpatient clinic with the belief that she was receiving special signs from the newspapers telling her that she had been singled out to perform a mission to save the world, and had started hearing voices telling her how to carry out her mission. She agrees that some of what has happened to her may be a trick of her mind, but not all. She agrees with you that she might be having a nervous breakdown, but is unwilling to come into hospital. What features would make hospital admission advisable and what features would make you content to treat her as an outpatient?

1.    Features indicating hospital admission:

- Ideas of self-harm or harm to others
- High levels of distress
- Impairment of nutrition
- Inadequate social support:

    i.    Social isolation, poor relationship with family, high expressed emotion, carers at the end of their tether or unable to contain the patient

- Community resources lacking

    i.    Inadequate number of community psychiatric nurses for example

- Reluctance to cooperate with treatment:

    i.    Previous history of non-cooperation as outpatient, lack of insight

- Excessive social stress
- Concomitant physical or psychiatric pathology that might complicate treatment and thus require a greater degree of supervision
- Assessment unclear:

    i.    For example, whether the patient really has a sleep disturbance.

2. Treatment at home:
   - Good social support:
     i. Living with understanding relatives/helpful neighbours
   - Non-urgent nature of the consultation
   - Assessment has excluded physical complications.

*What needs to be included in providing treatment at home?*

## What needs to be included in providing treatment at home?

1.  Assessment of the patient.

2.  Treatment:
    *   Provision of a neuroleptic drug
    *   Advice about potential side-effects and what to do if they occur
    *   Support from the community psychiatric nurse for the patient and the family/other carers
    *   Support/treatment at a day hospital or day centre (NB overstimulation may be an aggravating factor)
    *   Attention to aggravating factors
    *   Psychologist/family therapist if high expressed emotion
    *   Attention to financial/accommodation stressors.

3.  Monitoring:
    *   Regular appointments with psychiatrist, GP, community psychiatric nurse, social worker.

4.  Review/reassessment:
    *   When acute phase is over, devise longer term treatment plan.

# Further Reading

Creed F, Black D, Anthony P, Osborn M, Thomas P, Tomenson B (1990) Randomised controlled trial of day patient versus inpatient psychiatric treatment. *Br Med J* **300**: 1033–7

Groves T (1990) After the asylums. series *Br Med J* **300**:
The future of community care: 923–4
Who needs long-term psychiatric care? 999–1001
What does community care mean now? 1060–2
The local picture: 1128–30
Can the community care? 1186–8

Johnstone EC (1993) Schizophrenia — problems in clinical practice. *Lancet* **341**: 536–8

Melzer D, Hale AS, Malik SJ, Hogman GA, Wood S (1991) Community care for patients with schizophrenia one year after hospital discharge. *Br Med J* **303**: 1023–6

Muijen M, Marks IM, Conolly J, Audini B, McNamee G (1992) The Daily Living Programme — Preliminary comparison of community versus hospital-based treatment for the seriously mentally ill facing emergency admission. *Br J Psychiatry* **160**: 379–84

Thornicroft G, Bebbington P (1989) Deinstitutionalization — from hospital closure to service development. *Br J Psychiatry* **155**: 739–53

Tooth GC, Brook E M (1961) Trends in the mental hospital population and their effect on future planning. *Lancet* **i**: 710–3

Tyrer P, Turner R, Johnson AL (1989) Integrated hospital and community psychiatric services and use of inpatient beds. *Br Med J* **299**: 298–300

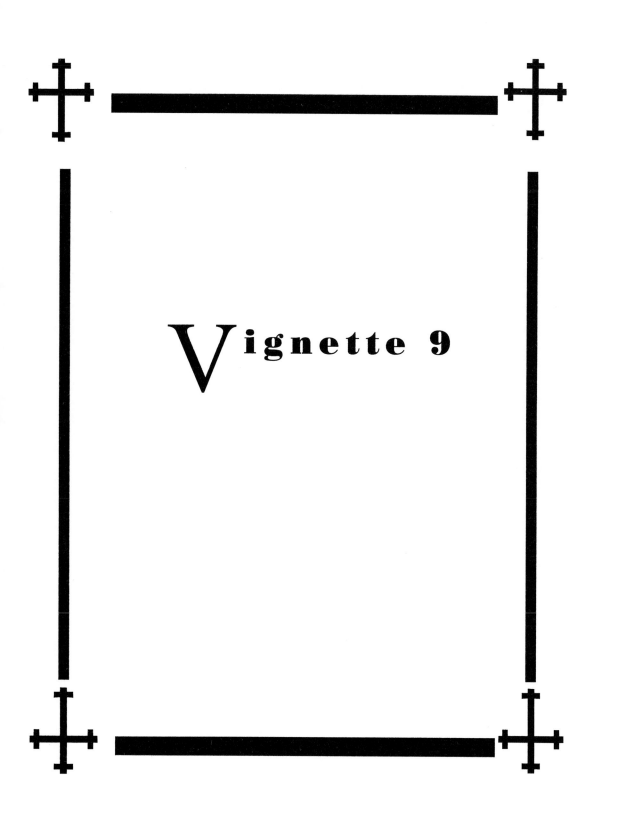

Vignette 9

# Vignette 9

You are called by the accident and emergency officer to see a 17-year-old man who was admitted the previous day following an overdose. How do you assess the severity of his overdose attempt from the history?

**You are called by the accident and emergency officer to see a 17-year-old man who was admitted the previous day following an overdose. How do you assess the severity of his overdose attempt from the history?**

1. Look for evidence that the patient meant to die:

   - Planning of the attempt
   - Tidying up of affairs

      i. Making a will, paying off of bills

   - Suicide note
   - Taking steps to ensure that he/she would not be found after the attempt:

      i. Going to a lonely/deserted/isolated place; carrying out the attempt when it was likely that no-one else would be around

   - Using a method that the patient thought was likely to be successful:

      i. If the patient thinks that four temazepam tablets are likely to be fatal, for example

   - Using a violent method:

      i. Hanging, shooting, jumping from a building or train.

2. Look for evidence of mental illness and try to understand whether the desire to commit suicide arose out of psychopathology

   - Depression
   - Schizophrenia
   - Personality disorder

*How do you assess continuing suicide risk?*

## How do you assess continuing suicide risk?

1.    Assess presence of treatable mental illness.

2.    Assess presence of suicidal intent (from patient and informants):
      - Does the patient regret that the overdose did not succeed in killing him?
      - Does he still think about killing himself?
      - Does he plan to make another suicide attempt?
      - If so, has he a detailed plan about how he will carry it out?
      - Has he made any attempt to harm himself while in hospital?

3.    Assess the level of his social support:
      - Will he be returning to a supportive and understanding family or does he live alone?
      - Will anything have changed in the social situation, or will he be returning to a situation likely to precipitate another suicide attempt?

*Having assessed the patient, you decide that he does not present a serious risk of another acute suicide attempt. You feel that he has a mild underlying depressive illness and could be followed up adequately by his GP. What initial advice would you give to the GP?*

Having assessed the patient, you decide that he does not present a serious risk of another acute suicide attempt. You feel that he has a mild underlying depressive illness and could be followed up adequately by his GP. What initial advice would you give to the GP?

1.    Consider an antidepressant drug:

    ● Preferably safe in overdose (e.g. lofepramine, a selective serotonin reuptake inhibitor (SSRI)).

2.    Ensure adequate dosage:

    ● Amitriptyline 150 mg/day equivalent.

3.    Give limited supply of tablet:

    ● For example, 7 days supply at a time.

4.    Review weekly for at least the first 4 weeks.

5.    After illness has remitted, continue antidepressant mdication in full doses for another 6 months.

6.    Re-refer if the situation deteriorates.

# Further Reading

Appleby L, Warner R (1993) Parasuicide; features of repetition and the implications for intervention. *Psychol Med* **23**: 13–16

Barraclough B, Bunch J, Nelson B, Sainsbury P (1974) 100 cases of suicide: clinical aspects, *Br J Psychiatry*, **125**: 355–73

Cassiday S, Henry J (1987) Fatal toxicity of antidepressant drugs in overdose. *Br Med J* **295**: 1021–4

Checkley S (1985) Biological markers in depression. In: Granville-Grossman K, ed. *Recent Advances in Clinical Psychiatry. Churchill Livingstone, London: 5*

Deakin JFW, ed. (1986) *The Biology of Depression.*. Gaskell, London

Gelder MG (1985) Cognitive therapy. In: Granville-Grossman K, ed. *Recent Advances in Clinical Psychiatry*. Churchill Livingstone, London: 5

Goldacre M, Seagroatt V, Hawton K (1993) Suicide after discharge from psychiatric inpatient care. *Lancet* **342**: 283–6

Hawton K, Catalan J (1981) Psychiatric management of the attempted suicide patients *Br J Hosp Med* **25**(4): 365–70

Isacsson G, Holmgren P, Wasserman D, Bergman U (1994) Use of antidepressants in people committing suicide in Sweden. *Br Med J* **308**: 506–9

Little JD (1992) Staff response to inpatient and outpatient suicide: what happened and what do we do? *Aus N Z J Psychiatry* **26**: 162–7

Medical Research Council (1965) Clinical trial of treatment of depressive illness; report to the Medical Research Council by its Clinical Psychiatry Committee. *Br Med J* **1**: 881–6

Morgan HG (1992) Suicide prevention. Hazards on the fast lane to community care *Br J Psychiatry* **160**: 149–53

O'Donnell I, Farmer R, Catalan J (1993) Suicide notes. *Br J Psychiatry* **163**: 45–8

Paykel ES, Coppen A, eds. (1979) *Psychopharmacology of Affective Disorders*. Oxford University Press, Oxford

Wexler BE, Cicchetti DV (1992) The outpatient treatment of depression — implications of outcome research for clinical practice *J Nerv Ment Dis* **180**: 277–86

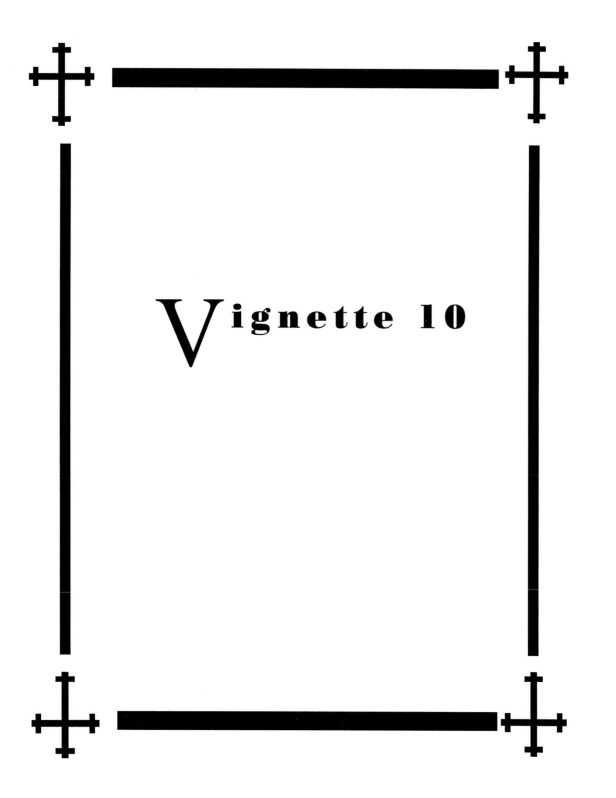

# Vignette 10

# Vignette 10

*You are asked to visit a hostel for people with learning disabilities where you are told that a 27-year-old man has become very disturbed and smashed a window. The staff are worried about him. When you arrive at the hostel, you are told that the man is giggling and saying "Thud" before laughing again. How do you handle the situation?*

You are asked to visit a hostel for people with learning disabilities where you are told that a 27-year-old man has become very disturbed and smashed a window. The staff are worried about him. When you arrive at the hostel, you are told that the man is giggling and saying "Thud" before laughing again. How do you handle the situation?

1.  Interview the staff and any other informant (including other residents):

    ● Find out exactly what happened
    ● Carry out a situational analysis:

        i.    Antecedents, behaviour, consequences

    ● Look at previous notes to find out:

        i.    Has this happened before?

        ii.   What happened then?

2.  Interview the patient:

    ● Try to understand both verbal and non-verbal communications
    ● Take a history and carry out a mental state examination as far as possible.

*What is the differential diagnosis?*

## What is the differential diagnosis?

- Acute distress (perhaps for an appropriate reason)

- Learned maladaptive behaviour

- Acute psychotic episode.

How might you diagnose schizophrenia or bipolar disorder in a person with learning difficulties?

# How might you diagnose schizophrenia or bipolar disorder in a person with learning difficulties?

1. Schizophrenia:
   - Deterioration from previous level of functioning
   - Irrational behaviour out of character
   - Evidence of hallucinations, although this may be poorly formed.

2. Hypomania:
   - Overactivity
   - Giggling
   - Disinhibition.

3. Depression:
   - Psychomotor retardation
   - Loss of appetite
   - Sleep disturbance
   - Lack of interest in things in which the person was normally interested.

What aspects of management should be considered in an acute psychotic episode in a person with learning difficulties?

## What aspects of management should be considered in an acute psychotic episode in a person with learning difficulties?

- A temporal epileptic focus may be contributing to the schizophrenia-like appearance

- Neuroleptic drugs are epileptogenic and should be used with particular caution in patients with known epilepsy

- Anticonvulsant medication, especially carbamazepine, may be useful, although lithium is still a first-line drug in the treatment of bipolar affective disorder.

# Further reading

Anonymous (1987) Management of behaviour problems in children with mental handicap. *Lancet* **i**: 545–6

Binfield SL (1992) Behaviour disorder in children and adolescents. *Curr Opin Psychiatry* **5**: 645–9

Fleisher MH (1991) Psychiatric disorder in adults. *Curr Opin Psychiatry*, **4**: 699–702

Fleisher MH (1992) Psychiatric disorder in adults. *Curr Opin Psychiatry* **5**: 668–71

Lindsey MP (1991) Behaviour disorder in children and adolescents. *Curr Opin Psychiatry* **4**: 693–8

Zigler E, Hodapp RM (1986) *Understanding Mental Retardation*. Cambridge University Press, Cambridge

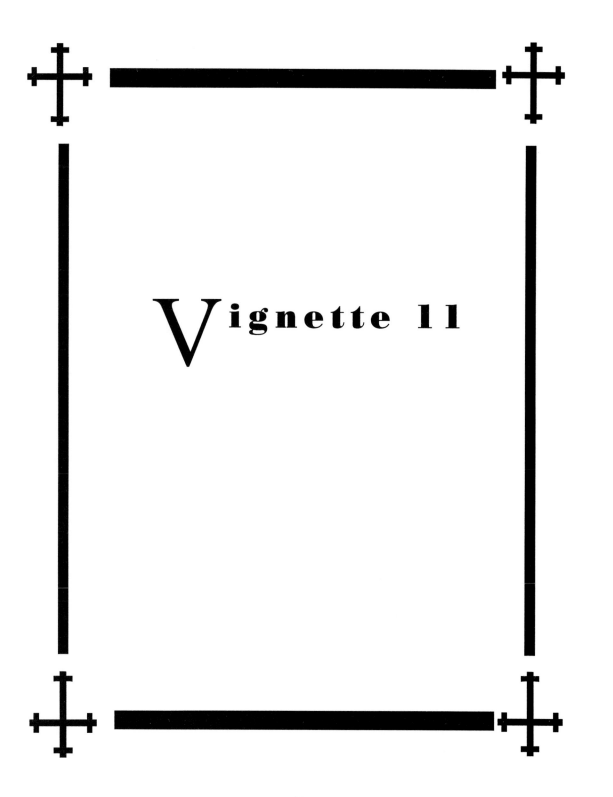

# Vignette 11

**Caution: this vignette deals with legal aspects of psychiatry and has been prepared by a practicing psychiatrist. The answers given here are in accordance with current psychiatric practice and, although every effort has been taken to ensure accuracy in law, they do not represent legal advice. If in doubt about the situation, proper legal advice should be sought from a duly qualified lawyer.**

# Vignette 11

*A GP rings to ask for your advice about a 47-year-old woman with a 25-year history of schizophrenia who is refusing treatment for a breast lump that the GP is convinced is malignant. Her husband feels that she should undergo mastectomy to save her life and wants to give consent on his wife's behalf. Can he do this?*

A GP rings to ask for your advice about a 47-year-old woman with a 25-year history of schizophrenia who is refusing treatment for a breast lump that the GP is convinced is malignant. Her husband feels that she should undergo mastectomy to save her life and wants to give consent on his wife's behalf. Can he do this?

No.

English law does not allow one person to give consent on behalf of another.

*In that case, could she not be compelled to have the operation under the Mental Health Act 1983, and if not, why not?*

## In that case, could she not be compelled to have the operation under the Mental Health Act 1983, and if not, why not?

No.

Part IV (Section 56–64) of the Mental Health Act 1983 which talks of Consent to Treatment specifies that it is applicable for medical treatment for mental disorder.

The *Code of Practice* (Department of Health and Welsh Office, 1993) states:

> `16.5 Part IV of the Act applies only to medical treatment for mental disorder. Treatment for physical disorder therefore cannot be given under this part of the Act unless it is a physical disorder that gives rise to a mental disorder and it is necessary to treat the physical disorder in order to treat the mental disorder.'*

*But if she's mad, she surely isn't in her right mind to be able to give consent. Can't we just do the operation anyway?*

**But if she's mad, she surely isn't in her right mind to be able to give consent. Can't we just do the operation anyway?**

Certainly not. Apart from the disrespectful and ignorant approach to mental illness on the part of the questioner, this has now been tested in law.

In the case re C (see Eastman (1994) `Further Reading), a man with a long-term history of schizophrenia developed gangrene. Although it was advised that if he did not undergo amputation of his leg he would die, he made the decision that he would rather die with both legs. The judge in the case upheld his capacity to give consent, saying that capacity to give consent was based on three factors:

- The ability to comprehend the nature of the medical problem
- The ability to weigh up the advantages and disadvantages
- The ability to form a belief.

Further discussion on capacity to consent to treatment can be found in Chapter 15 of the *Code of Practice* (Department of Health and Welsh Office 1993), noting that it was written before the case mentioned above went to law.

*So what do I do with this woman? Leave her to die?*

## So what do I do with this woman? Leave her to die?

1.  Ask for a psychiatric assessment:

    - It may be that she is refusing treatment because she has some delusionary belief about her medical illness or its treatment (e.g. she believes that she is God and can cure herself), in which case it would be appropriate to treat her mental illness (admitting her compulsorily to mental hospital if necessary), and then review her consent to treatment of her medical condition in the light of her improved mental state.

2.  Ensure that she has enough information on which to base her decision about whether to accept or refuse medical treatment:

    - this may involve the GP seeing the woman several times to give her support, encouragement to consider treatment, and repetition or further explanation of the medical reasons why treatment is highly advisable.

# Further reading

Brahams D (1988) A psychiatrist's duty of confidentiality (case of W). *Lancet* **ii**: 1503–4

Department of Health and Welsh Office (1993) *Code of Practice — Mental Health Act 1983.* Published August 1993 pursuant to section 118 of the Act. HMSO, London

Dyer C (1993a) Law Commission suggests help for mentally incapable. *Br Med J* **306**: 606

Dyer C (1993b) New law proposed for treatment mentally incapacitated people. *Br Med J* **306**: 1226

Eastman N (1994) Mental Health Law: civil liberties and the principle of reciprocity. *Br Med J* **308**: 43–5 (see letters on 5 February 1994, 408–9)

*Mental Health Act* 1983, HMSO: London

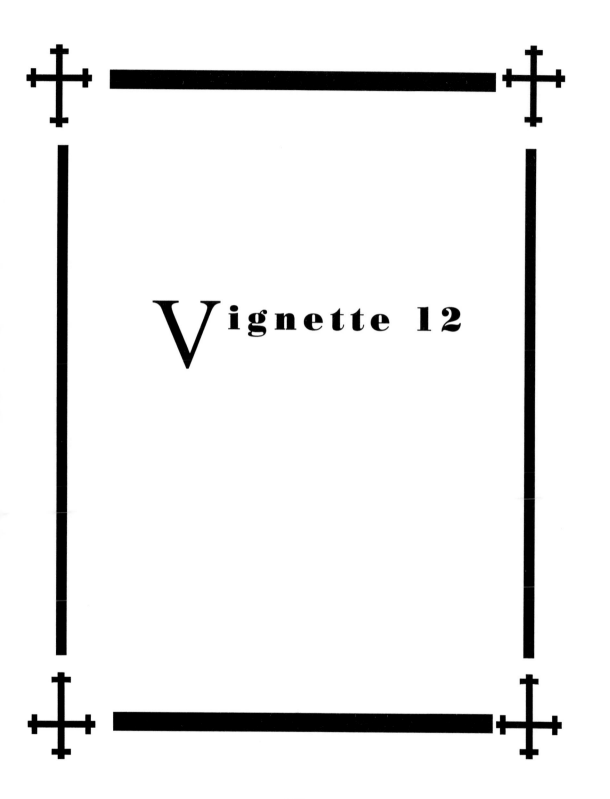

# Vignette 12

# Vignette 12

*For the last 3 years, your service has been monitoring a 24-year-old married woman who has a diagnosis of schizophrenia and has remained well on her depot neuroleptic medication. She attends a routine outpatient appointment accompanied by her husband to whom she has been happily married for 2 years, saying that she would like to become pregnant and start a family. She and her husband are seeking your advice about whether to go ahead with this course of action. What information do they need to know to help them decide?*

For the last 3 years, your service has been monitoring a 24-year-old married woman who has a diagnosis of schizophrenia and has remained well on her depot neuroleptic medication. She attends a routine outpatient appointment accompanied by her husband to whom she has been happily married for 2 years, saying that she would like to become pregnant and start a family. She and her husband are seeking your advice about whether to go ahead with this course of action. What information do they need to know to help them decide?

1.    Genetics:

The baby would have a greater risk of developing schizophrenia in his/her adult life than a baby born to parents who did not have schizophrenia, increasing from 1 to 12 % (i.e. it is 12 times greater, but there is an 8/10 chance that the baby will not develop schizophrenia [Fish's schizophrenia]).

2.    Her own illness.

She will probably be quite well during pregnancy, but there is a risk that she might relapse after the birth (puerperal psychosis).

They should consider whether they would be able to look after the baby when it is born. Factors that need attention would include:

- The extent of negative symptoms, which might impair her ability to perform child-rearing tasks for the child
- The strength of her social network: will another person (e.g. her mother or her husband) be around enough to provide a high level of support for the child?
  - i.    It is necessary to make some assessment of the likelihood of the social service department taking an interest in the welfare of the baby and the probability that it would be placed on the 'at risk' register or even be taken into care
- The presence of hallucinations and/or delusions that may be dangerous (e.g. delusions that she is evil) and any evidence of previously acting on delusions/hallucinations
- Her compliance with treatment and her responsiveness to neuroleptic medication.

The ultimate decision rests with the prospective parents and not the psychiatrist, whose role is to assist where possible with whichever decision the parents take

*They are worried that her current medication will harm the baby. How do you advise them and how do you manage her pregnancy from the psychiatric point of view?*

**They are worried that her current medication will harm the baby. How do you advise them and how do you manage her pregnancy from the psychiatric point of view?**

1.  Medication advice:

    ● While it is desirable that no medication should be prescribed in the first trimester, it will still have to be prescribed if there is risk of serious relapse (e.g. suicidal behaviour)

    ● Evidence suggests that the risk of teratogenicity from neuroleptic drugs in the first trimester is rare

    ● Nevertheless, ensure that she is maintained on the lowest dose consistent with maintenance of her mental state.

2.  Management of pregnancy:

    ● Ensure good liaison with the obstetric service and her general practitioner:

        i.   Good communication about the nature of her mental disorder and how it might affect her presentation to them

        ii.  Support and advice to obstetric medical and nursing staff if she develops a medical complication of pregnancy (e.g. advice about management of her neuroleptic medication; advice about accepting her without stigma and supporting her if she needs admission on to the obstetric ward)

        iii. Ensure that they understand the nature of her symptoms when psychiatrically ill and what to look out for in the puerperium as indicators of relapse so that advice may be sought quickly

        iv.  Ensure that steps will be taken to contact the psychiatric service and clear information about facilities (e.g. psychiatric mother-and-baby unit) is available

    ● Monitor her mental state closely during pregnancy
    ● Make particular efforts to alleviate or minimise psychosocial stressors that might precipitate relapse
    ● Should the situation change and it becomes likely that social services will recommend that the baby be taken from the mother, help needs to be given

to both parents so that they can come to terms with this unpleasant eventuality

## Further Reading

Appleby L (1991) Suicide during pregnancy and the first postnatal year. *Br Med J* **302**: 137–40

Appleby L, Fox H, Shaw M, Kumar R (1989) The psychiatrist in the obstetric unit: establishing a liaison service. *Br J Psychiatry* **154**: 510–5

Oates M (1989) Management of major mental illness in pregnancy and the puerperium. *Bailliere's Clin Obstet Gynaecol* **3**: 905–20

Sandler M (1978) *Mental Illness in Pregnancy and the Puerperium*. Oxford University Press, Oxford

Watson JP (1984) Psychiatric disorder in pregnancy and the first postnatal year. *Br J Psychiatry* **144**: 453–62

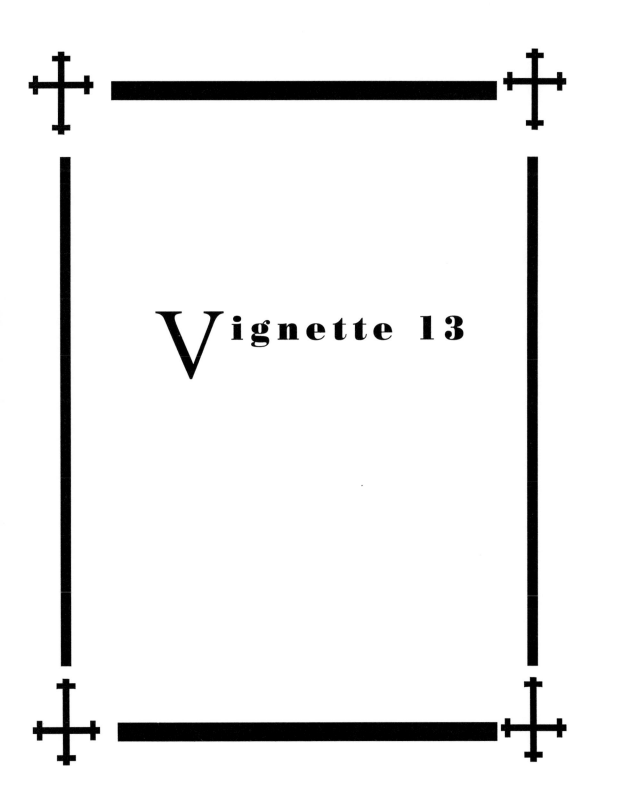

# Vignette 13

# Vignette 13

*A 59-year-old woman comes to the outpatient clinic with a history of bipolar affective disorder going back to the age of 22 years with several admissions to hospital, but has not been admitted for the last 10 years, having been well on lithium. However, one year previously, when she was being followed-up in the outpatient clinic, it was noticed that her urea and creatinine levels were rising, and you are now being asked to review her. How would you manage the situation?*

A 59-year-old woman comes to the outpatient clinic with a history of bipolar affective disorder going back to the age of 22 years with several admissions to hospital, but has not been admitted for the last 10 years, having been well on lithium. However, one year previously, when she was being followed-up in the outpatient clinic, it was noticed that her urea and creatinine levels were rising, and you are now being asked to review her. How would you manage the situation?

- Repeat a creatinine clearance test

- If there is evidence that her creatinine clearance has not declined, consider continuing lithium, but monitoring her carefully in the outpatient clinic with further creatinine clearance tests on a regular basis (e.g. annually)

- If there is evidence that her creatinine clearance has declined, consider changing her medication from lithium to carbamazepine.

*Four months after her creatinine clearance tests showed a decline in renal function, lithium was discontinued and carbamazepine started. She returns to the outpatient clinic with a 3 week history of depressed mood, sleeping only 2 hours a night, constipation and finding everything an effort, with no motivation. How do you manage the situation now?*

**Four months after her creatinine clearance tests showed a decline in renal function, lithium was discontinued and carbamazepine started. She returns to the outpatient clinic with a 3 week history of depressed mood, sleeping only 2 hours a night, constipation and finding everything an effort, with no motivation. How do you manage the situation now?**

1.   Assess the extent of her depressive mood state, paying particular attention to suicidal ideation and nutrition.

2.   Although stopping lithium is the most likely cause for relapse in this patient, do not forget to search for other possible precipitants.

3.   Check her carbamazepine level and adjust carbamazepine dose accordingly.

4.   Consider adding an antidepressant drug:
   - This is a matter of balancing risks and benefits
   - Use a low dose initially (e.g. 75 mg/day imipramine equivalent)
   - Monitor frequently watching for precipitation into hypomania.

5.   Consider location of treatment:
   - Day hospital admission may be helpful, although a place may not be readily available
   - Inpatient admission may be considered, but given the non-urgent nature of the case may be unnecessary
   - Management may be in the outpatient department if there is adequate social support from the family. A community psychiatric nurse may prove helpful in monitoring the patient's clinical state.

# Further reading

Elphick M (1989) The use of carbamazepine in psychiatry. *Psychol Med* 19: 591–604

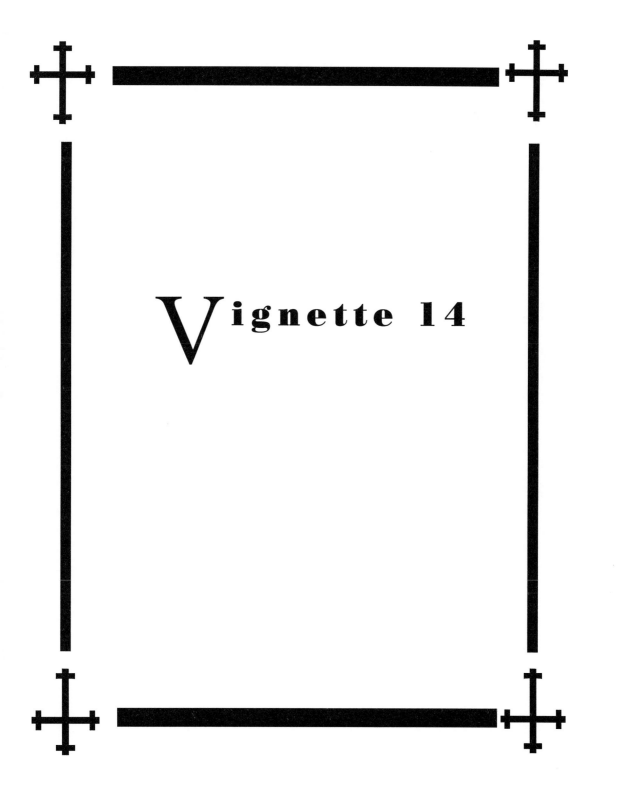

# Vignette 14

# Vignette 14

*A 53-year-old man was admitted to the ward 6 weeks ago after being brought in by his wife who said that she had found him in the kitchen with a knife, saying that he was going to kill himself. Examination had shown him to have depressed mood and he was saying that he wanted to kill himself because he realised that he should be punished for having stolen a bag of sweets from a shop 7 years ago and, that morning, voices had told him to kill himself. He agreed to come into hospital to please everyone, but felt deep down that there was no point as his life was soon coming to an end. He had not been a management problem in that he stayed on the ward and took his prescribed medication of amitriptyline 150 mg at night, with no ill effects. Nevertheless, 6 weeks later he is no better. What therapeutic strategies are open to you?*

A 53-year-old man was admitted to the ward 6 weeks ago after being brought in by his wife who said that she had found him in the kitchen with a knife, saying that he was going to kill himself. Examination had shown him to have depressed mood and he was saying that he wanted to kill himself because he realised that he should be punished for having stolen a bag of sweets from a shop 7 years ago and, that morning, voices had told him to kill himself. He agreed to come into hospital to please everyone, but felt deep down that there was no point as his life was soon coming to an end. He had not been a management problem in that he stayed on the ward and took his prescribed medication of amitriptyline 150 mg at night, with no ill effects. Nevertheless, 6 weeks later he is no better. What therapeutic strategies are open to you?

- Change to another antidepressant drug, e.g. another tricyclic, a selective serotonin reuptake inhibitor (SSRI), or a monoamine oxidase inhibitor (MAOI)

- Add lithium

- Administer electroconvulsive therapy (ECT).

*The notes from another hospital arrive as you are trying to choose between the therapeutic options, and show that he was admitted there 10 years ago with a similar picture and had a very long admission. Three different antidepressant drugs (two different tricyclics and a monoamine oxidase inhibitor (MAOI)) were tried in adequate doses for adequate periods of time without any benefit, but he had responded promptly to electroconvulsive therapy (ECT). He is agreeable to a course of ECT, for which his wife had been clamouring for the last 2 weeks. You decide that ECT may be worth considering. What are the clinical indications for ECT?*

The notes from another hospital arrive as you are trying to choose between the therapeutic options, and show that he was admitted there 10 years ago with a similar picture and had a very long admission. Three different antidepressant drugs (two different tricyclics and a monoamine oxidase inhibitor (MAOI)) were tried in adequate doses for adequate periods of time without any benefit, but he had responded promptly to electroconvulsive therapy (ECT). He is agreeable to a course of ECT, for which his wife had been clamouring for the last 2 weeks. You decide that ECT may be worth considering. What are the clinical indications for ECT?

- Psychotic depression

- Catatonia

- Agitated depression

- Acute, severe neuroleptic-resistant mania.

*How do you choose between unilateral and bilateral electrode placement?*

### How do you choose between unilateral and bilateral electrode placement?

- Memory impairment is less with unilateral ECT

- Bilateral ECT is a more powerful antidepressant treatment.

# Further reading

Letemendia FJJ, Delva M, Rodenburg M *et al* (1993) Therapeutic advantages of bifrontal electrode placement in ECT. *Psychol Med* **23**: 349–60

Linington A, Harris B (1988) Fifty years of electroconvulsive therapy. *Br Med J* **297**: 1354–5

The Royal College of Psychiatrists (1977) Memorandum on the use of electroconvulsive therapy. *Br J Psychiatry* **131**: 261–72

The Royal College of Psychiatrists' ECT Subcommittee of the Research Committee (1989) *The Practical Administration of Electroconvulsive Therapy (ECT)*. Gaskell, London

Scott AIF (1994) Contemporary practice of ECT. *Br J Hosp Med* **51**: 334–9

Zielinski RJ, Roose SP, Devanand DP, Woodring S, Sackeim HA (1993) Cardiovascular complications of ECT in depressed patients with cardiac disease. *Am J Psychiatry* **150**: 904–9

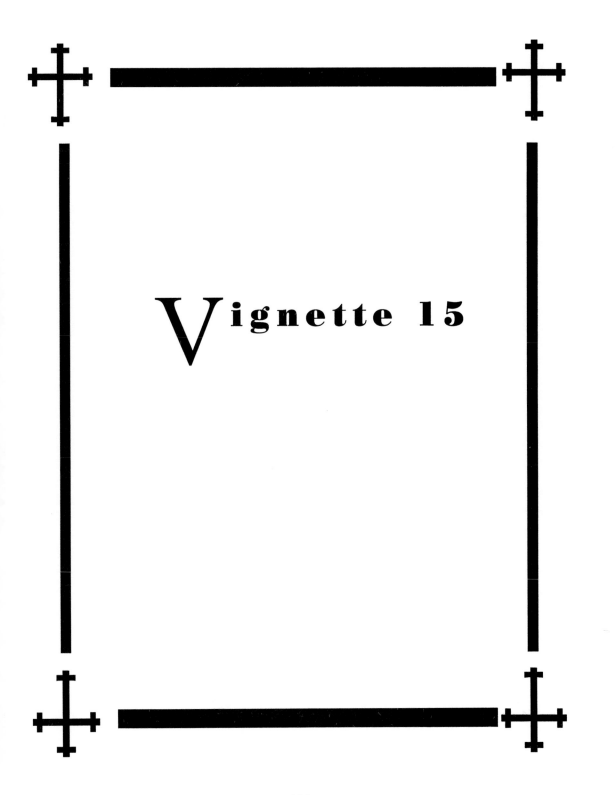

Vignette 15

# Vignette 15

*A 45-year-old businessman is referred for the first time to a psychiatrist by the GP because he is depressed. Although work is stressful, the business is ticking over nicely. There are no domestic problems, nor has he had any recent life events. The GP says that the only past medical history was an endoscopy 3 years previously for epigastric pain that showed a normal gastro-intestinal tract, recent full physical examination was unremarkable and he is taking no prescribed medication of any sort. What is the most important potential contributory factor still needing to be excluded?*

A 45-year-old businessman is referred for the first time to a psychiatrist by the GP because he is depressed. Although work is stressful, the business is ticking over nicely. There are no domestic problems, nor has he had any recent life events. The GP says that the only past medical history was an endoscopy 3 years previously for epigastric pain that showed a normal gastro-intestinal tract, recent full physical examination was unremarkable and he is taking no prescribed medication of any sort. What is the most important potential contributory factor still needing to be excluded?

●     Alcohol

*After taking a full alcohol history, it emerges that he has been drinking heavily during his working life, with business lunches being an important part of his work. What features make you think that he might be chemically dependent on alcohol?*

After taking a full alcohol history, it emerges that he has been drinking heavily during his working life, with business lunches being an important part of his work. What features make you think that he might be chemically dependent on alcohol?

1.    Withdrawal symptoms:

- Retching, sweating, shaking
- History of delirium tremens, epileptic fits.

2.    A history of the alcohol dependence syndrome:

- Narrowing of the drinking repertoire, subjective awareness of a compulsion to drink, repeated withdrawal symptoms, salience of drink-seeking behaviour, increased tolerance to alcohol, relief drinking, reinstatement after abstinence.

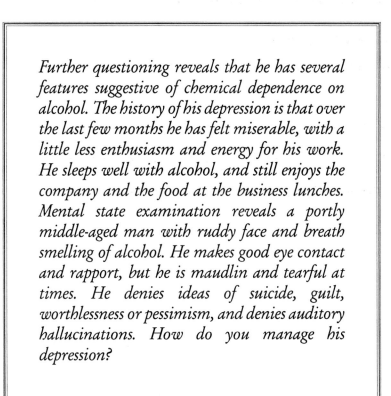

*Further questioning reveals that he has several features suggestive of chemical dependence on alcohol. The history of his depression is that over the last few months he has felt miserable, with a little less enthusiasm and energy for his work. He sleeps well with alcohol, and still enjoys the company and the food at the business lunches. Mental state examination reveals a portly middle-aged man with ruddy face and breath smelling of alcohol. He makes good eye contact and rapport, but he is maudlin and tearful at times. He denies ideas of suicide, guilt, worthlessness or pessimism, and denies auditory hallucinations. How do you manage his depression?*

Further questioning reveals that he has several features suggestive of chemical dependence on alcohol. The history of his depression is that over the last few months he has felt miserable, with a little less enthusiasm and energy for his work. He sleeps well with alcohol, and still enjoys the company and the food at the business lunches. Mental state examination reveals a portly middle-aged man with ruddy face and breath smelling of alcohol. He makes good eye contact and rapport, but he is maudlin and tearful at times. He denies ideas of suicide, guilt, worthlessness or pessimism, and denies auditory hallucinations. How do you manage his depression?

1.  The mood should, ideally, be assessed when he is not inebriated:

    ● First he should undergo inpatient or outpatient detoxification.

2.  Repeat physical examination/blood tests in case of physical cause for low mood.

3.  Repeat/intensify search for psychosocial factors, with informant history.

4.  If in doubt, consider an antidepressant drug, even in the absence of biological symptoms. Alcoholics have a much higher incidence of suicide. Because of this, choose an antidepressant drug that is unlikely to be dangerous in overdose, e.g. a selective serotonin reuptake inhibitor (SSRI).

5.  Offer help and advice to keep the patient off alcohol:
    ● AA, Accept, Alcohol Recovery Project
    ● Motivational interviewing
    ● Cognitive–behavioural therapy
    ● Stress management
    ● Disulfiram/calcium carbimide.

# Further reading

Edwards G (1982) *The Treatment of Drinking Problems*. Grant McIntyre, London

Edwards G, Gross MM (1976) Alcohol dependence: provisional description of a clinical syndrome. *Br Med J* i: 1058–61

Madden JS (1993) Alcohol and depression. *Br J Hosp Med* 50: 261–4

Miller WR, Rollnick WR (1991) *Motivational Interviewing*. Guilford Press, New York

Mueller TI, Lavori PW, Keller MB *et al* (1994) Prognostic effect of the variable course of alcoholismon the 10-year course of depression. *Am J Psychiatry* 151: 701–6

Royal College of Psychiatrists (1986) *Alcohol — Our Favourite Drug*. Tavistock, London

Shuckit MA, Monteiro MG (1988) Alcoholism, anxiety and depression. *Br J Addict* 83: 1373–80

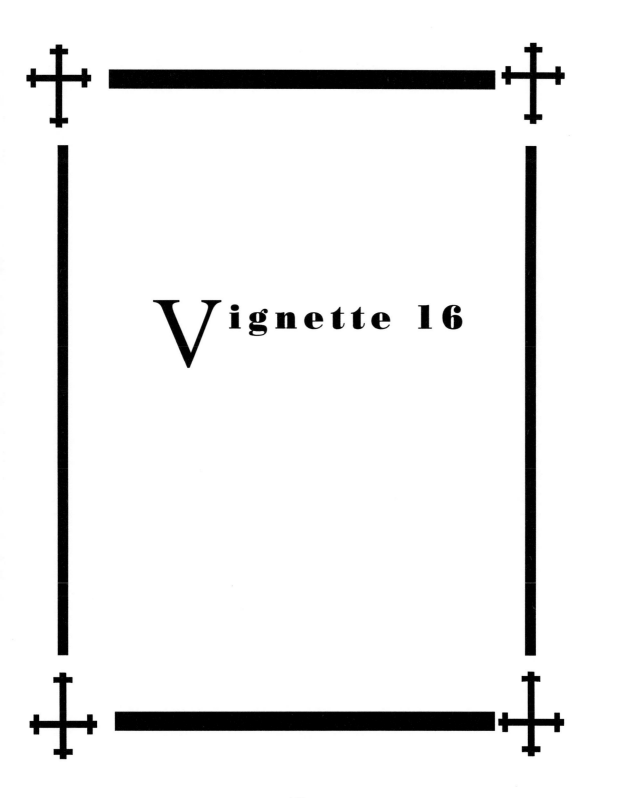

# Vignette 16

# Vignette 16

*Your secretary informs you that she has been called by the local prison medical officer to say that a remand prisoner who has been living in your catchment area has been behaving strangely, expressing paranoid ideas and has been refusing food. What is the procedure for going to see him in prison and how do you carry out this assessment?*

**Your secretary informs you that she has been called by the local prison medical officer to say that a remand prisoner who has been living in your catchment area has been behaving strangely, expressing paranoid ideas and has been refusing food. What is the procedure for going to see him in prison and how do you carry out this assessment?**

1.   Ring up the prison hospital office and make an appointment:

   •   You will not be allowed in unless the staff at the main gate of the prison have been informed that you are an expected official visitor

   •   The time will most likely be limited to within office hours (including the time by which the visit must be completed).

2.   Be on time, and make sure that you have evidence of personal identification.

3.   When you arrive, you may be asked to go through a metal detector.

4.   You will be met by a prison nursing officer who will escort you to the hospital wing.

5.   It is reasonable to ask to see the prison hospital medical notes. These may provide helpful information and observations. Prison medical/nursing staff may be reluctant to let you see these notes if you are engaged by the defence solicitor, but it is reasonable to point out to them that this will limit your examination, to the detriment of both patient and the legal process.

6.   Ensure that you know the nature of the charges against the patient and the likely consequences (especially whether a conviction could lead to a prison sentence).

7.   Ensure that you are clear about what is being asked of you:

   •   An immediate assessment of the patient's mental health

   •   An assessment of the mental state of the patient at the time of the alleged crime

   •   An admission to your hospital (in which case ask yourself if you have the resources to care for the patient securely)

   •   A court report.

8.   Ask to see any other documents relating to the case:

* For example, statements of other witnesses.

9.   Ask to see the patient in private in an appropriate room:

* However, you may have a prison nursing officer in the room with you if you have reason to believe that it would not be safe to be alone with the prisoner.

10.  Explain to the prisoner the nature of the assessment, including the fact that although you will do everything you can to respect confidentiality, as an expert witness you may be required to reveal information that you have been given to the court. In light of this, the patient may refuse to confide in you.

11.  Remember your role as an expert witness:

* It is not your role to sympathise or act as an advocate for the client (the solicitor and barrister are employed to present the client in the most favourable light)
* Neither is it your role to condemn the patient (the judge and jury can decide the patient's guilt)
* It is your role to assess the patient impartially and use your expert knowledge as a psychiatrist to elucidate any factors that:

    i.   Suggest the patient did or did not have a mental illness that required treatment

    ii.  Have a bearing on the appropriateness of convicting the patient

    iii. Have a bearing on his disposal.

12.  Make sure that you make detailed contemporaneous notes, including the length of time spent with the patient, the names and jobs/relationship to the patient of those whom you interviewed directly, and the documents that you read in relation to the case.

*After your initial assessment, you determine that the patient is suffering from mental illness and requires hospital admission. What is the legal process for this in the case of a prisoner on remand?*

**After your initial assessment, you determine that the patient is suffering from mental illness and requires hospital admission. What is the legal process for this in the case of a prisoner on remand?**

Section 48 of the Mental Health Act 1983 empowers the Secretary of State, on the recommendations of two registered medical practitioners, to give a transfer direction in respect of someone suffering from mental illness or severe mental impairment of a nature or degree which makes it appropriate for him to be detained in hospital for medical treatment and who is in urgent need of such treatment.

(Section 35 allows for a remand to hospital for a report on an accused's mental condition.)

*Your assessment revealed that the patient assaulted a neighbour with a hammer because he believed that the neighbour had been playing music loudly to annoy him. The patient knew this because he could hear the neighbour's son shouting through the walls "We'll get you, you pig". History from the neighbour reveals her to be childless. There is a history of admission to two other psychiatric hospitals following disputes with neighbours before the patient moved into your catchment area. What recommendations might you make to the court?*

Your assessment revealed that the patient assaulted a neighbour with a hammer because he believed that the neighbour had been playing music loudly to annoy him. The patient knew this because he could hear the neighbour's son shouting through the walls "We'll get you, you pig". History from the neighbour reveals her to be childless. There is a history of admission to two other psychiatric hospitals following disputes with neighbours before the patient moved into your catchment area. What recommendations might you make to the court?

You might recommend that the patient is suffering from schizophrenia and that an appropriate disposal would be to admit him to your hospital under section 37 of the Mental Health Act 1983.

If the court accepts your basic recommendation about the mental health of the patient but is concerned about potential dangers, the court may also choose to add a restriction order under section 41 of the Mental Health Act 1983.

*The court takes your advice and the patient is transferred to your acute admission ward. There, he cooperates with treatment and makes no attempt to abscond, developing quite a good rapport with the staff. How do you manage him?*

**The court takes your advice and the patient is transferred to your acute admission ward. There, he cooperates with treatment and makes no attempt to abscond, developing quite a good rapport with the staff. How do you manage him?**

As with any other patient suffering from an acute relapse of schizophrenia, paying special attention to:

- Neuroleptic medication:

    i.    After obtaining his cooperation, he will probably require depot medication over a period of years

    ii.   Ensure extra awareness of the development of side-effects such as parkinsonism and tardive dyskinesia, as these will make his necessary treatment less acceptable

    iii.  Pay added attention to titration of dose

- Aftercare planning (needs to be careful and detailed):

    i.    Keyworker identification and initiation of relationship

    ii.   Housing:

          *In view of what happened to his neighbour, he may well not be able to return to his former abode and may require re-housing*

    iii.  Occupation

    iv.   Emotional support during the transition back to the community and help in re-establishing old social networks or developing new ones.

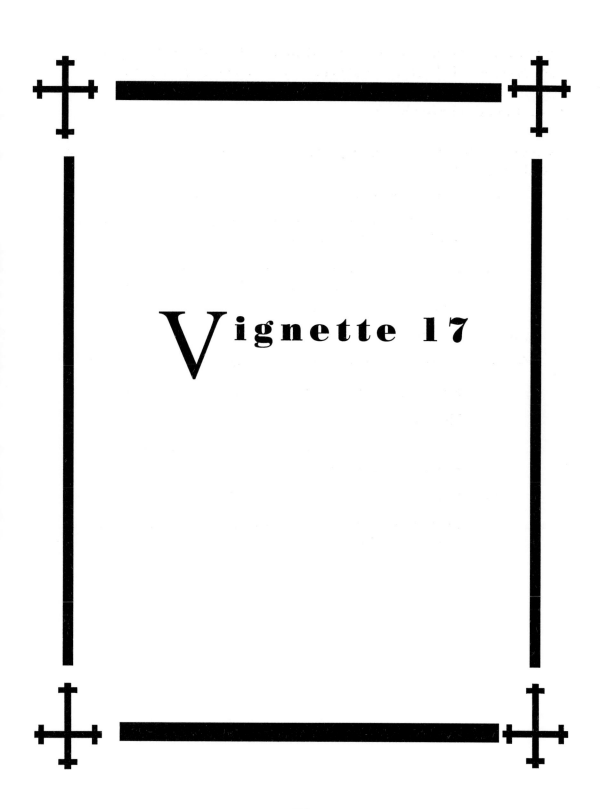

# Vignette 17

# Vignette 17

A 56-year-old man is sent to your outpatient clinic because he is depressed. He says that he has been married to his wife for the last 29 years and although it has been a good marriage, he feels miserable because he thinks that she has started to have an affair. For 2 years, his wife has undertaken a part-time job as a sales assistant in a department store, and he feels certain that she has started `carrying on' on with one of the men at work, although he has not yet found proof. As a result, they have been rowing more frequently. His own life is in the doldrums because his company is having difficulties, and it is uncertain whether the factory is going to close. Orders are sluggish and although redundancy is a possibility, no decision has been made. He feels unmotivated to work and easily argues with his wife. What is the differential diagnosis?

A 56-year-old man is sent to your outpatient clinic because he is depressed. He says that he has been married to his wife for the last 29 years and although it has been a good marriage, he feels miserable because he thinks that she has started to have an affair. For 2 years, his wife has undertaken a part-time job as a sales assistant in a department store, and he feels certain that she has started 'carrying on' with one of the men at work, although he has not yet found proof. As a result, they have been rowing more frequently. His own life is in the doldrums because his company is having difficulties, and it is uncertain whether the factory is going to close. Orders are sluggish and although redundancy is a possibility, no decision has been made. He feels unmotivated to work and easily argues with his wife. What is the differential diagnosis?

- 'Mid-life crisis'

- Neurotic depression

- Morbid jealousy

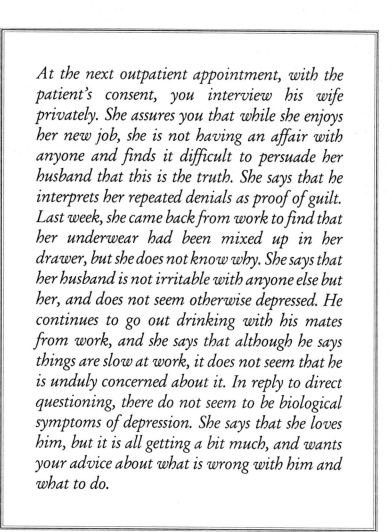

*At the next outpatient appointment, with the patient's consent, you interview his wife privately. She assures you that while she enjoys her new job, she is not having an affair with anyone and finds it difficult to persuade her husband that this is the truth. She says that he interprets her repeated denials as proof of guilt. Last week, she came back from work to find that her underwear had been mixed up in her drawer, but she does not know why. She says that her husband is not irritable with anyone else but her, and does not seem otherwise depressed. He continues to go out drinking with his mates from work, and she says that although he says things are slow at work, it does not seem that he is unduly concerned about it. In reply to direct questioning, there do not seem to be biological symptoms of depression. She says that she loves him, but it is all getting a bit much, and wants your advice about what is wrong with him and what to do.*

At the next outpatient appointment, with the patient's consent, you interview his wife privately. She assures you that while she enjoys her new job, she is not having an affair with anyone and finds it difficult to persuade her husband that this is the truth. She says that he interprets her repeated denials as proof of guilt. Last week, she came back from work to find that her underwear had been mixed up in her drawer, but she does not know why. She says that her husband is not irritable with anyone else but her, and does not seem otherwise depressed. He continues to go out drinking with his mates from work, and she says that although he says things are slow at work, it does not seem that he is unduly concerned about it. In reply to direct questioning, there do not seem to be biological symptoms of depression. She says that she loves him, but it is all getting a bit much, and wants your advice about what is wrong with him and what to do.

1. Morbid jealousy is the probable diagnosis.

2. The prognosis for the disorder is poor, but may be containable if he takes neuroleptic medication regularly.

3. In this disorder, there is a real risk of the patient harming his wife, and she should consider leaving him if:

   - He becomes increasingly irritable or the frequency of rows increases
   - He refuses to take medication
   - He refuses to attend outpatient appointments
   - He increases his alcohol intake
   - He makes threats to harm or kill her; such threats should always be taken seriously in this disorder.

# Further reading

Bishay NR, Petersen N, Tarrier N (1989) An uncontrolled study of cognitive therapy for morbid jealousy. *Br J Psychiatry* **154**: 386–9

Enoch MD, Trethowan WH (1979) The Othello syndrome. In: Enoch MD, Trethowan WH, eds. *Uncommon Psychiatric Syndromes.* 2nd edn. John Wright, Bristol

Shepherd M (1961) Morbid jealousy: some clinical and social aspects of a psychiatric symptom. *J Ment Sci* **107**: 687–705

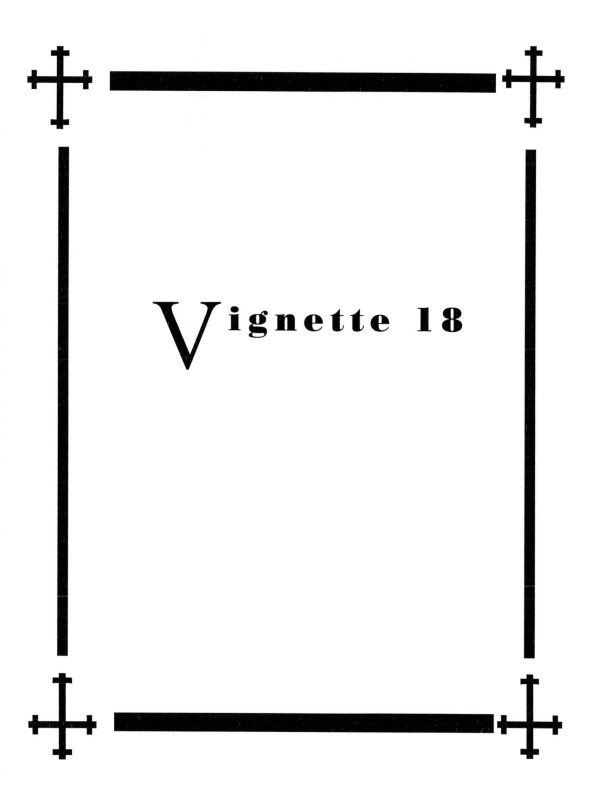

# Vignette 18

# Vignette 18

*A community psychiatric nurse contacts you to say that one of her patients who has a diagnosis of schizophrenia, and whom she has been seeing for over a year to give him his depot medication, is now saying that he wants to stop the depot medication. How do you manage the situation?*

A community psychiatric nurse contacts you to say that one of her patients who has a diagnosis of schizophrenia, and whom she has been seeing for over a year to give him his depot medication, is now saying that he wants to stop the depot medication. How do you manage the situation?

1.  See the patient, preferably with the community psychiatric nurse present to avoid splitting; i.e. Setting two people (in this case two professionals) against each other by telling them different things.

2.  Review the notes:
    - What were the original symptoms?
    - How many previous episodes has the patient had?
    - How long did they last?
    - How easily did the symptoms respond to the reintroduction of neuroleptic medication?

3.  Examine the patient's mental state:
    - If stable, stopping the depot medication may be an option
    - If not, you will have to be firm in your advice not to stop medication.

4.  Find out the reason why the patient wants to stop now:
    - He never was happy taking medication in the first place, and this is just another request of many to stop
    - His mental state is stable, and he feels that he no longer needs to take medication
    - He has developed side-effects
    - He would prefer to take the medication orally.

*On seeing the patient, he is adamant that he is well and does not need any more medication. His mother with whom he lives reminds you that he is fine as long as he takes his medication, but becomes unwell if he does not. She asks if he could be given the depot medication against his will under the Mental Health Act 1983. The patient makes it clear that he is not going to accept the next injection. How do you manage the situation?*

On seeing the patient, he is adamant that he is well and does not need any more medication. His mother with whom he lives reminds you that he is fine as long as he takes his medication, but becomes unwell if he does not. She asks if he could be given the depot medication against his will under the Mental Health Act 1983. The patient makes it clear that he is not going to accept the next injection. How do you manage the situation?

1. If his mental state does not warrant compulsory admission, he cannot be given treatment against his will in the community:

   - R v Hallstrom (1985) (see Brahams 1986) makes it clear that admitting a patient overnight under section 3, giving him depot medication and then putting him on long leave is not legal if its real purpose is to give compulsory treatment in the community

   - The legal mechanism of a Community Treatment Order has been requested by the Royal College of Psychiatrists, but has not, at present, been accepted by the Government.

2. Schizophrenia does not deprive the patient of learning capacity, and he is as able to respond to a behavioural approach as is someone without schizophrenia. Thus he can be allowed to make choices, but be aware that he will not be spared the consequences of those choices:

   - He may become unwell again
   - He may require admission earlier than if he continued to take the medication
   - If he has a further psychotic episode, he may not return to his former level of functioning despite reinstatement of treatment
   - His family have the right to cease to look after him at any time, and the ability and/or willingness of his family to do so may be decreased by his unwillingness to continue adequate treatment.

3.  Having made a change of treatment plan which includes stopping his medication, plans must be made for his continuing care:

    - Establish that the community psychiatric nurse is prepared to remain the key worker

    - Establish that his family are prepared to continue to care for the time being or refer to a social worker for rehousing

    - Clarify what the early symptoms of relapse are likely to be, and make sure that these are clearly documented and well-known to all who are involved in his care

    - Ensure that all who might be involved in his care are promptly informed of the change of plan, especially the GP

    - Establish a system to monitor his mental state, e.g. regular visits by the community psychiatric nurse, regular outpatient review — this may not have to be frequent

    - Ensure that the system can respond if a deterioration in his mental state is noted:

        i.   The work telephone numbers of professionals involved in his care should be readily available

        ii.  There should be ease of access to information concerning the patient for a duty doctor or duty social worker if called outside normal working hours, including a written plan for relapse, such as early admission.

# Further reading

Brahams D (1986) Treatment of unco-operative psychiatric patients in the community: Mental Health Act in need of reform. *Lancet* **i**: 863–4

Coid J (1994) Failure in community care: psychiatry's dilemma. *Br Med J* **308**: 805–6

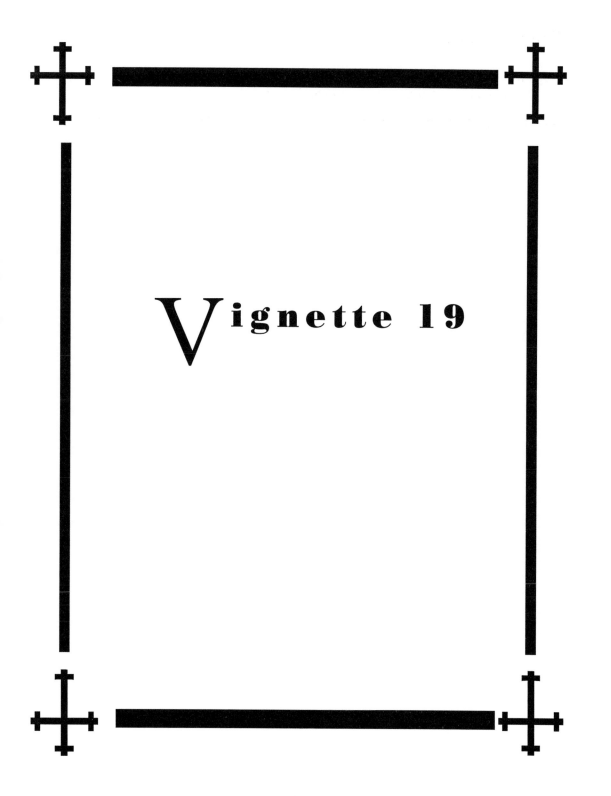

Vignette 19

# Vignette 19

*A 34-year-old man with schizophrenia who is reasonably well, controlled on his depot neuroleptic medication, attends the outpatient department with his wife. She says that she has recently noticed that her husband has been making strange movements with his mouth, and she wonders what they might be. What is the differential diagnosis?*

A 34-year-old man with schizophrenia who is reasonably well, controlled on his depot neuroleptic medication, attends the outpatient department with his wife. She says that she has recently noticed that her husband has been making strange movements with his mouth, and she wonders what they might be. What is the differential diagnosis?

1.  Disorders arising out of schizophrenia:

    - A disease-related dyskinesia
    - A movement that he is making in response to some other psychopathology, e.g. an auditory hallucination.

2.  A disorder as a side-effect of neuroleptic treatment:

    - Drug-induced Parkinsonism
    - Tardive dyskinesia.

3.  Non-psychiatric disorders:

    - Neurological disorders
    - Dental problems.

*What are the risk factors for tardive dyskinesia?*

## What are the risk factors for tardive dyskinesia?

- Older age

- Female sex

- Neuroleptic medication being used for a condition other than schizophrenia, e.g. affective psychosis

- Organic brain damage

- Addition of anticholinergic agent

- Early Parkinsonism

- Acute dystonia

- Acute akathisia.

*How do you manage tardive dyskinesia?*

## How do you manage tardive dyskinesia?

1. Prevention:

   • Try to prevent it occurring and watch for it in follow-up of patients:

      i. Careful initial prescription

      ii. Continue neuroleptic medication only if the patient is benefitting

      iii. Use the minimum dose possible for clinical efficacy

      iv. Avoid drug holidays

      v. Avoid anticholinergic medication where possible

      vi. Use caution in patients with affective disorder or brain damage.

1. Once the patient is suffering from tardive dyskinesia:

   • If neither the patient nor the relative are concerned, it may be appropriate to do nothing

   • Evaluate risks and benefits:

      i. It may be worth accepting the disadvantage of tardive dyskinesia for the benefit of non-relapse into a very damaging psychotic episode

   • There is no satisfactory pharmacological strategy, but there are several possible alternative strategies:

      i. Increase the dose of the neuroleptic drug, although this may set up a vicious cycle

      ii. Slow, stepwise dimunition of neuroleptic medication

      iii. Stop anticholinergic medication if possible

      iv. Pharmacological strategies include:

      *Cholinergics*

      *Physostigmine, choline, lecithin, deanol*

      *Gamma aminobutyric acid mimetics*

*Benzodiazepines (diazepam, clonazepam)*

*Baclofen, sodium valproate, muscimol*

*Low-dose dopamine agonists — to reduce supersensitivity*

*Apomorphine, L-dopa, bromocriptine*

*Calcium channel blockers*

*Verapamil, diltiazem*

*Lithium*

*Manganese*

*Propranolol*

*α-Tocopherol*

*Electroconvulsive therapy*

- Stopping the neuroleptic drug, if possible, may be followed by resolution. Tardive dyskinesia is not always irreversible, although drug holidays are associated with an increased risk of tardive dyskinesia.

## Further reading

Barnes TRE (1983) Tardive dyskinesia; a 3 year follow-up study. *Psychol Med* **13**: 71–81

Barnes TRE (1988a) Tardive dyskinesia. *Br Med J* **296**: 150–1

Barnes TRE (1988b). Tardive dyskinesia: risk factors, pathophysiology and treatment. In: Granville-Grossman K, ed. *Recent Advances in Clinical Psychiatry.* Churchill Livingstone, London

*Drugs and Therapeutics Bulletin* (1986) Management of tardive dyskinesia. *Drug Ther Bull* **24**: 27–8

Jeste DV (1979) Tardive dyskinesia: reversible and persistent. *Arch Gen Psychiatry* **36**: 585

Klawans HL, Goetz CG, Perlik S (1980) Tardive dyskinesia: review and update. *Am J Psychiatry* **137**: 900–8

Task Force (1980) Tardive dyskinesia: summary of an APA task force report. *Am J Psychiatry* **137**: 163–72

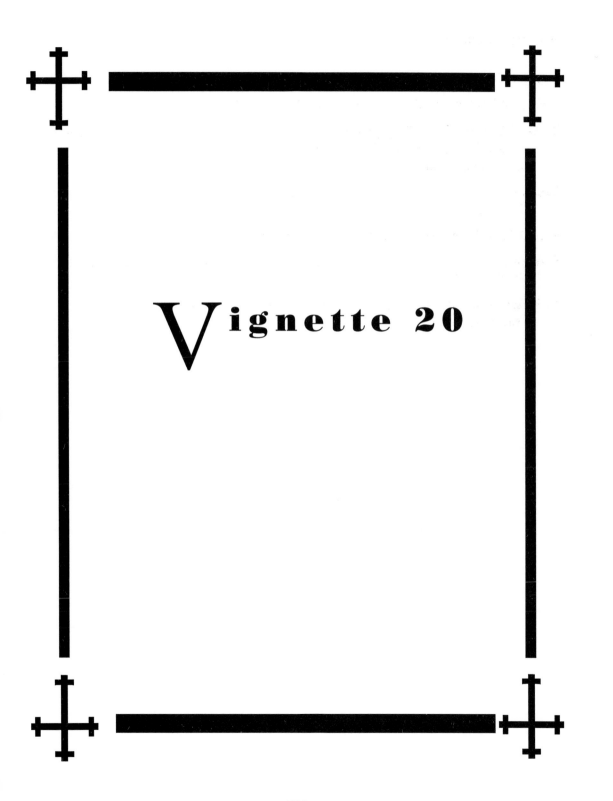

# Vignette 20

# Vignette 20

*A 37-year-old man comes to see you complaining of depression. He says that he has felt depressed since he was a teenager, but that 4 days ago he had smashed up his flat following an argument with his girlfriend. Since then he has felt even more unhappy, cannot be bothered to eat, is finding nothing of interest and is thinking of taking his own life. What is the differential diagnosis at this stage?*

A 37-year-old man comes to see you complaining of depression. He says that he has felt depressed since he was a teenager, but that 4 days ago he had smashed up his flat following an argument with his girlfriend. Since then he has felt even more unhappy, cannot be bothered to eat, is finding nothing of interest and is thinking of taking his own life. What is the differential diagnosis at this stage?

- Acute reaction to stress

- Depressive illness

- Personality disorder

*What questions would you ask to determine whether he had an antisocial personality disorder?*

## What questions would you ask to determine whether he had an antisocial personality disorder?

1.    What was he like at school?

   - Look for evidence of truanting, bullying others, being expelled or suspended from school, leaving school early without qualifications.

2.    What is his occupational record?

   - Look for evidence of many changes of job, each of short duration; evidence associated with being sacked for poor timekeeping or leaving abruptly following an argument with the boss; and evidence of long periods of unemployment.

3.    What is his drug history?

   - Look for evidence of the use of benzodiazepines, sometimes in high doses, to deal with feelings of tension; look for evidence of illicit drug use.

4.    What is his alcohol use?

   - This may be excessive either because of his social groupings or to deal with feelings of tension.

5.    What is his forensic history?

   - Look for convictions of assault of others and damage to property.

6.    What is his psychosexual history?

   - Look for many brief relationships, perhaps with violence in the relationship.

*Further history reveals that he has had several episodes of violence to property, and has been to prison on two occasions for assault. He has a poor work record, failing to stay in a job longer than 2 or 3 days. He is threatened with an injunction not to see his girlfriend, whom he has beaten up on many occasions. He expresses some concern about his tendency to violent outbursts and wants help. What can you offer?*

Further history reveals that he has had several episodes of violence to property, and has been to prison on two occasions for assault. He has a poor work record, failing to stay in a job longer than 2 or 3 days. He is threatened with an injunction not to see his girlfriend, whom he has beaten up on many occasions. He expresses some concern about his tendency to violent outbursts and wants help. What can you offer?

1.   Medication:

   ● Sometimes neuroleptic medication or lithium have been found helpful.

2.   Day hospital/outpatient support.

3.   Anger management programmes:

   ● If they are available.

4.   Supportive psychotherapy/keyworker:

   ● Regular sessions to deal with coping in general
   ● Early or urgent sessions to deal with crises, both practical and feelings of anger and suicidality.

5.   Social worker advice:

   ● He may need help with practical problems, such as rehousing and benefits, and support in dealing with the frustrations inherent in the system, e.g. the slow speed with which this help may be obtained or difficulties in communication with the staff with whom he comes in contact.

# Further reading

Lewis A (1974) Psychopathic personality — a most elusive category. *Psychol Med* **4**: 133–40

Lewis G, Appleby L (1988) Personality disorder — the patients psychiatrists dislike. *Br J Psychiatry* **153**: 40–50

Siever LJ, Davis KL (1991) A psychobiological perspective on the personality disorders. *Am J Psychiatry* **148**: 1647–58

Stone MH (1993) Long-term outcome in personality disorders. *Br J Psychiatry* **162**: 299–313

Tyrer P, Ferguson B, Casey P (1991) Personality disorder in perspective. *Br J Psychiatry* **159**: 463–72

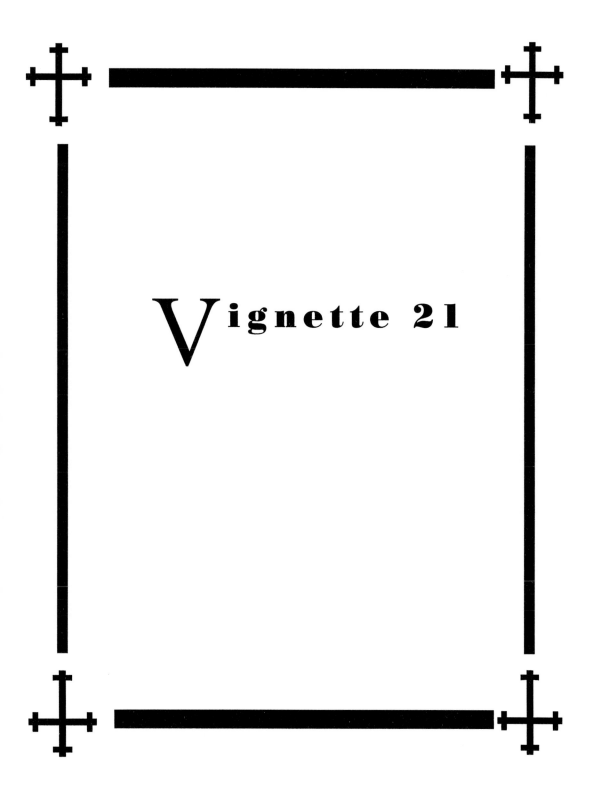

# Vignette 21

# Vignette 21

You are asked to assess a 24-year-old man with a psychiatric history for dangerousness. What points do you consider?

## You are asked to assess a 24-year-old man with a psychiatric history for dangerousness. What points do you consider?

There is no certain way of evaluating dangerousness at present, and it is self-deceptive for a psychiatrist to believe that he is capable of such an assessment.

However, psychiatrists are often asked to offer advice to courts, and certain points are worth bearing in mind.

1.    General.

    Violence predicts violence:

- Once a person has committed a violent act, he will find it easier to commit another.

    The violent act requires the sum of:

*Perpetrator + victim + location/situation*

- Is the perpetrator going to return to exactly the same situation in which he previously offended?

2.    Specifically psychiatric:

    Is there a psychiatric diagnosis, and if so is it relevant in this case?

- For example, a person with the alcohol dependence syndrome who is not motivated to stop drinking may have committed an offence when drunk. Apart from the fact that being drunk is not a defence to a crime, e.g. murder, such a person is likely to drink again and therefore is more likely to offend again.

    What was the mental state of the offender at the time of the offence?

- If the perpetrator committed a violent act when psychotic owing to a specific psychopathology, e.g. command hallucinations, then it may be reasonable to assume that the risk of dangerousness is greatly reduced if the patient is maintained in a relatively normal mental state by the use of medication, e.g. a neuroleptic drug.

- Therefore, consider:

    i.   Compliance of the patient with treatment

    ii.  Responsiveness to neuroleptic medication

    iii. Precipitants to psychosis in the social environment, e.g. high expressed emotion regarding the family.

For other points, see Scott(1977) in 'Further reading'.

*In the course of your interview, the patient tells you that he is having thoughts about murdering his girlfriend. He describes his plan in detail and then says that he has not told anyone else as they might try to stop him. He feels able to tell you as you are bound by your duty of confidentiality. How do you handle the situation?*

**In the course of your interview, the patient tells you that he is having thoughts about murdering his girlfriend. He describes his plan in detail and then says that he has not told anyone else as they might try to stop him. He feels able to tell you as you are bound by your duty of confidentiality. How do you handle the situation?**

You may want to discuss the situation with your professional defence adviser. He may advise you that there are times when a professional has a duty to act in the public interest in precedence to his duty of confidentiality to a client. In particular, he may cite:

- The Tarasoff case (see Bluglass 1979)
- The case of W (see Brahams 1988).

As a result of your discussions with your adviser, you may feel that the overriding concern should be to protect the girlfriend and that:

- She should be informed
- The judge should be informed and your advice about the disposal of the patient modified accordingly
- The doctor/psychiatrist in charge of the care of the patient should be informed.

If you remain the doctor in charge of the care of the patient, it will be necessary to discuss with him the fact that you cannot act as though he had not confided in you

- it may take some time to rebuild the trust between you

# Further reading

Bluglass R (1979) The psychiatric assessment of homicide. *Br J Hosp Med* **22**: 366–77

Brahams D (1988) A psychiatrist's duty of confidentiality (case of W). *Lancet* **ii**: 1503–4

Hamilton JR, Freeman H, eds (1982) *Dangerousness: Psychiatric Assessment and Management*. Gaskell, London

Mullan PE (1988) Violence and mental disorder. *Br J Hosp Med* **40** (6): 460–3

Scott PD (1977) Assessing dangerousness in criminals. *Br J Psych* **131**: 127–42

Taylor PJ, Gunn J (1984a) Violence and psychosis. I — Risk of violence among psychotic men. *Br Med J* **288**: 1945–9

Taylor PJ, Gunn J (1984b) Violence and psychosis. II — Effect of psychiatric diagnosis on conviction and sentencing of offenders. *Br Med J* **289**: 9–12

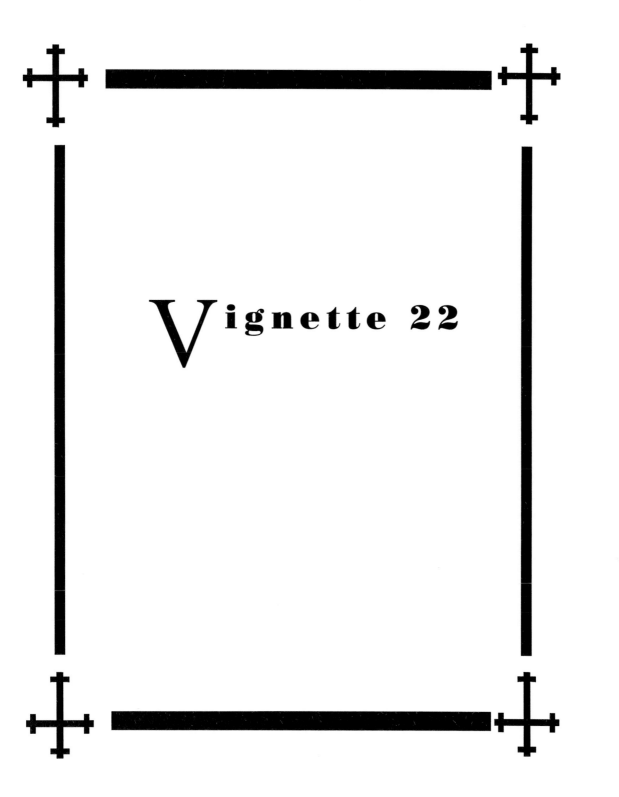

Vignette 22

# Vignette 22

*In the course of a team meeting, one of the nurses comments that a 45-year-old man with a diagnosis of schizophrenia who has been well controlled on a neuroleptic drug seems to be depressed at the moment. What is the differential diagnosis?*

**In the course of a team meeting, one of the nurses comments that a 45-year-old man with a diagnosis of schizophrenia who has been well controlled on a neuroleptic drug seems to be depressed at the moment. What is the differential diagnosis?**

1.    A deterioration in his schizophrenia.

2.    Depression superimposed on schizophrenia.

3.    Negative symptoms of schizophrenia.

4.    Iatrogenic causes:
    - Haloperidol, fluphenazine
    - So-called 'akinetic depression' (i.e. extrapyramidal side-effects).

5.    Undiagnosed physical illness:
    - Hypothyroidism
    - Drug-induced hepatitis.

6.    Concomitant alcoholism/drug abuse.

*Further enquiry of the nurse and examination of the patient reveal no psychosocial cause for this deterioration, nor any physical cause. He does not drink or misuse illicit drugs. What therapeutic options are open to you?*

Further enquiry of the nurse and examination of the patient reveal no psychosocial cause for this deterioration, nor any physical cause. He does not drink or misuse illicit drugs. What therapeutic options are open to you?

- Increase the dose of the neuroleptic drug

- Add an antidepressant drug

- Change the neuroleptic drug from one associated with depression to one that is not, e.g. flupenthixol

- Consider electroconvulsive therapy.

*List the negative symptoms of schizophrenia and say what you might do to treat them*

## List the negative symptoms of schizophrenia and say what you might do to treat them

1.  Symptoms:

    - Alogia
    - Affective flattening
    - Apathy
    - Anergy
    - Avolition
    - Anhedonia
    - Asociality
    - Attentional impairment.

2.  Management:

    - Stimulate the patient, encouraging him to be active:

        i.  Occupational therapy, activities, attendance at day hospital/sheltered workshop

    - Medication:

        i.  An alerting neuroleptic drug, such as flupenthixol, may be effective for anergy or anhedonia

        ii. Risperidone; clozapine is sometimes helpful.

# Further reading

Andreasen NC, Olsen S (1982) Negative v positive schizophrenia — definition and validation. *Arch Gen Psychiatry* **39**: 789–94

Barnes TRE, Curson DA, Liddle PF, Patel M (1989) The nature and prevalence of depression in chronic schizophrenic inpatients. *Br J Psychiatry* **154**: 486–91

House A, Bostock J, Cooper J (1987) Depressive syndrome in the year following onset of a first schizophrenic illness. *Br J Psychiatry* **151**: 773–9

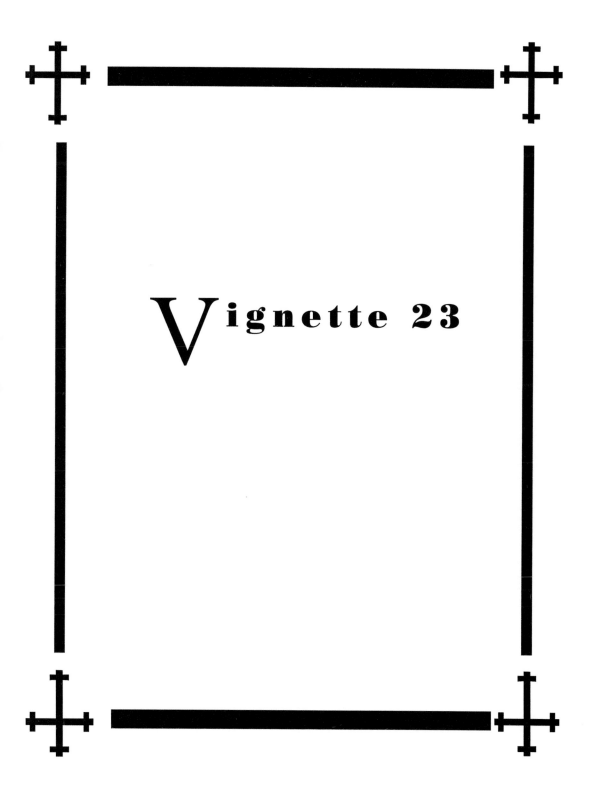

# Vignette 23

# Vignette 23

*A GP rings you to say that he has just seen a girl who came in complaining of `depression', but he thinks that she has anorexia nervosa, and wonders whether she needs to be acutely admitted as an inpatient. From his narration, you agree that the history, which includes anorectic attitudes, suggests anorexia nervosa as the probable diagnosis. What are the guidelines for further management?*

A GP rings you to say that he has just seen a girl who came in complaining of 'depression', but he thinks that she has anorexia nervosa, and wonders whether she needs to be acutely admitted as an inpatient. From his narration, you agree that the history, which includes anorectic attitudes, suggests anorexia nervosa as the probable diagnosis. What are the guidelines for further management?

Use the body mass index (BMI) to evaluate weight loss:

$$BMI = \frac{weight(kg)}{height(metres)^2}$$

Rules of thumb:

| | |
|---|---|
| *BMI 19–24* | *Normal* |
| *BMI 16–19* | *Outpatient treatment* |
| *BMI 13–16* | *Day hospital treatment* |
| *BMI < 13* | *Inpatient admission* |

(While these reflect work in a specialist Eating Disorder unit, the threshold for inpatient admission in a general hospital psychiatric unit might be at a slightly higher BMI.)

*What are anorectic attitudes?*

## What are anorectic attitudes?

1.  Preoccupation with body weight:
    - Distorted: perceived as being too fat
    - Size of cheeks, breasts, thighs, buttocks, abdomen.

2.  Preoccupation with food:
    - Concern about eating too much
    - Rumination:
        i.    Food is bad
        ii.   Calorific value of food
        iii.  What to select
        iv.   How to get rid of it.

3.  Preoccupation in cooking for others.

4.  Hiding, eating alone, food fads.

*Her BMI is 13.2, but you advise hospital admission. She agrees to come in as an informal patient. How do you manage her in hospital, and what advice do you give to the nurses about how to deal with her?*

**Her BMI is 13.2, but you advise hospital admission. She agrees to come in as an informal patient. How do you manage her in hospital, and what advice do you give to the nurses about how to deal with her?**

1. Ideally, only an identified group of members of staff will be involved in her management. In practice, this may not be possible.

2. Communication between staff needs to be as detailed as possible:

   - Patients with eating disorders tend to split staff frequently, and uncertainty about the current rules (e.g. whether she is allowed out of bed, allowed to leave half a potato) puts the staff member on duty in a difficult position
   - Because of well-meant sympathy for the patient, arguments between staff can easily arise, e.g. one member of staff may become an advocate for the patient against another. This needs to be dealt with promptly in order to prevent conflict and disunity among the staff, and because this dynamic is a means by which the patient can avoid dealing with her own illness.

3. Ensure that the plan of management is clear to the patient and to the staff:

   - The current plan should be clearly written
   - Unless there is an extremely good reason, the plan should be agreed and changed only at team meetings, with the agreement of the patient.

4. The overall plan for the complete admission should indicate a target weight for discharge and a realistic speed of weight gain, e.g. 1 kg/week:

   - It should also indicate when the patient will be weighed (twice weekly), on which scales — these should be of a high standard and constant — and what clothing should be worn
   - The patient should have constant feedback of her weight
   - Weight loss will be the best indication that she is still emotionally very distressed.

5. The weekly plan should contain details of:

   - Whether she is to be confined to bed/wear nightclothes
   - Whether she may have privileges, such as visitors or whether she may go off the ward

- What she is expected to eat (in consultation with a dietician), the length of time in which she should eat and whether she needs constant observation outside her supervised mealtimes (e.g. following to the toilet to prevent self-induced vomiting)
- A timetable of how she will spend her time during the week.

6.    Other aspects of her treatment on the ward might include:

- Regular weekly counselling with a constant staff member
- Body image therapy
- Group therapy if other patients with eating disorders are present
- Dynamic psychotherapy (if she is already seeing a therapist in the unit) can be resumed as her physical state improves
- Family therapy sessions
- Careful monitoring of her physical condition, especially her plasma potassium level
- Antidepressant medication where it is clear that low mood is not just secondary to starvation.

# Further reading

American Psychiatric Association (1993) Practice guidelines for eating disorders. *Am J Psychiatry* **150**: 207–28

Holden NL (1989) Eating disorders. *Bailliere's Clin Obstet Gynaecol 3(4): 705–27*

Hsu LKG (1986) The treatment of anorexia nervosa. *Am J Psychiatry* **143**: 573–81

Russell GFM, Szmukler GI, Dare C, Eisler I (1987) An evaluation of family therapy in anorexia nervosa and bulimia nervosa. *Arch Gen Psychiatry* **44**: 1047–56

Treasure J (1987) The biochemical and hormonal sequelae of the eating disorders. *Br J Hosp Med* **37**(4): 301–3

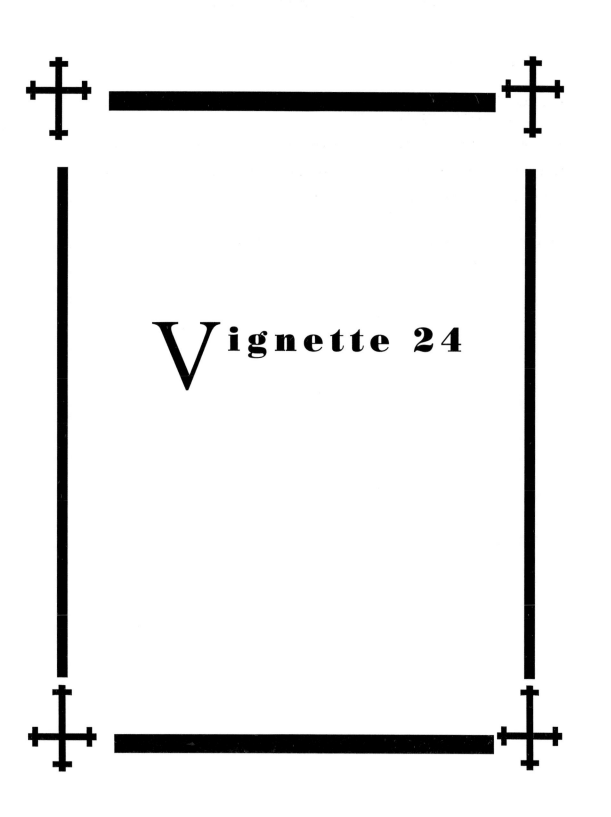

# Vignette 24

# Vignette 24

*An experienced marital therapist rings to ask you to see a 26-year-old woman. The therapist has been seeing her and her husband, and says that the patient complains of her husband being unreasonably impatient and angry with her, while her husband says that he gets frustrated because his wife is terribly slow about everything. You are being asked to see the woman because the situation seems to be getting the wife down, and the therapist is wondering if she is getting depressed. What might be happening?*

An experienced marital therapist rings to ask you to see a 26-year-old woman. The therapist has been seeing her and her husband, and says that the patient complains of her husband being unreasonably impatient and angry with her, while her husband says that he gets frustrated because his wife is terribly slow about everything. You are being asked to see the woman because the situation seems to be getting the wife down, and the therapist is wondering if she is getting depressed. What might be happening?

1.   There is an incompatibility in the relationship that may or may not be resolvable.

2.   The wife may have a psychiatric disorder:
   ● Depressive illness:
      i.   Primary depression
      ii.  Depression secondary to an underlying medical disorder, e.g. hypothyroidism, anaemia, Addison's disease, systemic lupus erythematosus, cancer
   ● Obsessional slowness
   ● Chronic fatigue syndrome
   ● Schizophrenia:
      i.   Either with negative symptoms or features of catatonia
   ● Substance abuse
      i.   Especially opiates or benzodiazepines.

3.   The husband may have an emotional or psychiatric disorder:
   ● He may have traits of intolerance, lack of consideration for others, or impatience
   ● Explosive personality
   ● Hypomania
   ● Thyrotoxicosis

- Substance abuse:

    i.  Especially alcohol or cocaine.

It is worth noting that when an experienced colleague in the mental health field refers an individual for investigation, they are usually correct and it would not be surprising that in the situation described in this vignette, the wife would be found to have a psychiatric disorder.

*On examination of the woman, she complains that her husband is always rushing her out of the house when they go out, and is not willing to wait while she checks that the taps and light switches are off and the doors are properly bolted. This leads to constant rows. What particular psychiatric diagnosis might you want to exclude; what questions would you ask and what answers would you expect if the diagnosis is present?*

On examination of the woman, she complains that her husband is always rushing her out of the house when they go out, and is not willing to wait while she checks that the taps and light switches are off and the doors are properly bolted. This leads to constant rows. What particular psychiatric diagnosis might you want to exclude; what questions would you ask and what answers would you expect if the diagnosis is present?

## Obsessive–compulsive disorder (OCD)

Questions might include:

1.  How long does it take you to get out of the house after you have checked everything?

    - An answer of more than a few minutes would be suspicious. In severe OCD, she might take 30 minutes to 1 hour or more.

2.  How many times do you have to check before you are satisfied that all is in order?

    - If she has to check more than once or twice, then it is probably pathological.

3.  Why do you check more than once?

    - If she has OCD, the patient will describe an obsessive thought, such as doubts about whether she did lock the front door coming into her head against her will and even when she knows that she did lock the door. She will try to resist these doubts, but will remain uncertain and become increasingly anxious until she tries to relieve the anxiety by checking again; a compulsive action.

*After completing the psychiatric examination, you conclude that she has OCD without any other psychiatric diagnoses. How do you manage her condition?*

**After completing the psychiatric examination, you conclude that she has OCD without any other psychiatric diagnoses. How do you manage her condition?**

With her permission, explain the diagnosis and the nature of the illness to both her and her husband.

1.  Drug treatment:

    - Clomipramine
    - Selective serotonin reuptake inhibitors.

2.  Behavioural treatment:

    - Exposure (systematic desensitisation)
    - Thought stopping
    - Homework assignments.

# Further reading

Drummond LM (1993) The treatment of severe, chronic, resistant obsessive–compulsive disorder. *Br J Psychiatry* **163**: 223–9

Tynes LL, White K, Steketee GS (1990) Towards a new nosology of obsessive–compulsive disorder. *Comp Psychiatry* **163**: 465–80

Veale D (1993) Classification and treatment of obsessional slowness. *Br J Psychiatry* **162**: 198–203

Zetin M, Kramer MA (1992) Obsessive–compulsive disorder. *Hosp Comm Psychiatry* **43**: 689–99

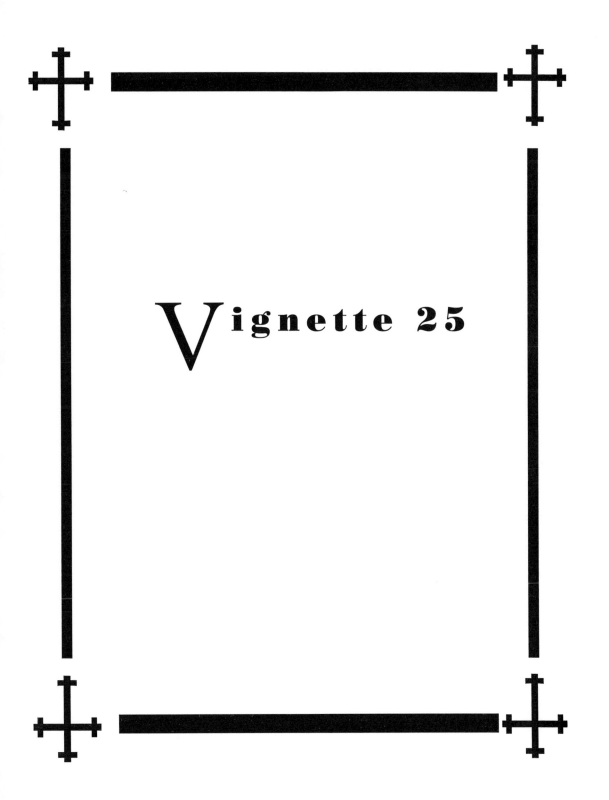

# Vignette 25

# Vignette 25

*You are sitting in the canteen at a table with a group of junior doctors. As they are leaving, a newly qualified surgical houseman 2 days into his first job remarks that he has just got the result of a biopsy for one of his patients. The result shows that the patient has a malignant growth and the houseman is dreading having to break the bad news. As he is talking, you realise that the others have left and that it is to you that he is talking. How do you advise him to break the bad news?*

You are sitting in the canteen at a table with a group of junior doctors. As they are leaving, a newly qualified surgical houseman 2 days into his first job remarks that he has just got the result of a biopsy for one of his patients. The result shows that the patient has a malignant growth and the houseman is dreading having to break the bad news. As he is talking, you realise that the others have left and that it is to you that he is talking. How do you advise him to break the bad news?

1. See the patient in private if possible.

2. Try and do so at a time when you can give him your full attention, and will not be disturbed:

   - Do not rush to tell him, or tell him in passing
   - If he asks for the results when you are rushed, tell him that you have some information but that you need to sit down and talk with him about it:

     i. Although you will be concerned that this would leave him worrying, it will allow him to prepare himself for the news that is to come.

3. When you are settled with him:

   - Tell him that you need to discuss his results
   - Watch for his response, both verbal and non-verbal:

     i. If he indicates that he does not want to know the truth, accept whatever untruth he wishes to believe and do not proceed, e.g. if he says something like "It's not serious is it, doctor? It's only an ulcer, isn't it?", do not disagree but be sympathetically non-committal and leave it. The patient will indicate at some later date if his state of mind has changed and he now feels able to cope with the truth, with some comment such as "Could we talk again, doctor? I know you said that it was an ulcer, but it's more than that, isn't it?"

     ii. If it appears that he does want to know more, he will not interrupt, or will indicate that you should proceed

   - Give a statement that the news is bad
   - When he seems able to take the information, use lay terminology without being brusque. Something like "You have a growth. It's not good". The

patient may well come out with "Is it cancer?", to which you can nod agreement sympathetically

- When the patient has had time to take in the information, answer any questions about the aetiology, management and prognosis that the patient asks
- When the interview seems to be finished, offer to discuss it again with the patient
- Ensure that the patient and his relatives are left with some time and space to express their emotion privately

4. Remember, it is the patient who has the right to the information, not the relatives:

- Do not accede to the relatives' wishes to keep him ignorant of the truth unless the patient himself indicates that he does not really wish to know the truth:

   i.   Keeping information from a patient who wishes to know his diagnosis at the request of his family makes the period of terminal illness harder for the patient and his family, not easier

- The patient is the one who has the right to inform others or keep it hidden from others. He should decide who will be with him when he is told, and whom he wishes you to talk to afterwards:

   i.   If he refuses to let you talk with anyone, you have no right to break that confidentiality, although it is appropriate to point out that the period of his terminal illness will be harder if he does choose to keep the diagnosis from those who are closest to him.

*Three months later, you bump into the same houseman again. He thanks you for your previous helpful advice, which was very effective. He now says that the patient, who seemed initially to take the information well, is moody and irritable. What might be happening to him and what advice would you give to the houseman?*

Three months later, you bump into the same houseman again. He thanks you for your previous helpful advice, which was very effective. He now says that the patient, who seemed initially to take the information well, is moody and irritable. What might be happening to him and what advice would you give to the houseman?

1.  Possible diagnoses:

    - The patient is grieving his own death
    - Depressive illness.

2.  Treatment options:

    - Grief counselling
    - Antidepressant medication
    - Electroconvulsive therapy if psychotic depression.

# Further reading

Maguire P (1988a) How to improve the counselling skills of doctors and nurses in cancer care. *Br Med J* **ii**: 847

Maguire P (1988b) How to communicate with cancer patients. 1. Handling bad news and difficult questions. *Br Med J* **ii**: 907

Maguire P (1988c) How to communicate with cancer patients. 2. Handling uncertainty, collusion and denial. *Br Med J* **ii**: 972

Maguire P (1994) ABC of breast diseases: psychological aspects. *Br Med J* **309**: 1649–52

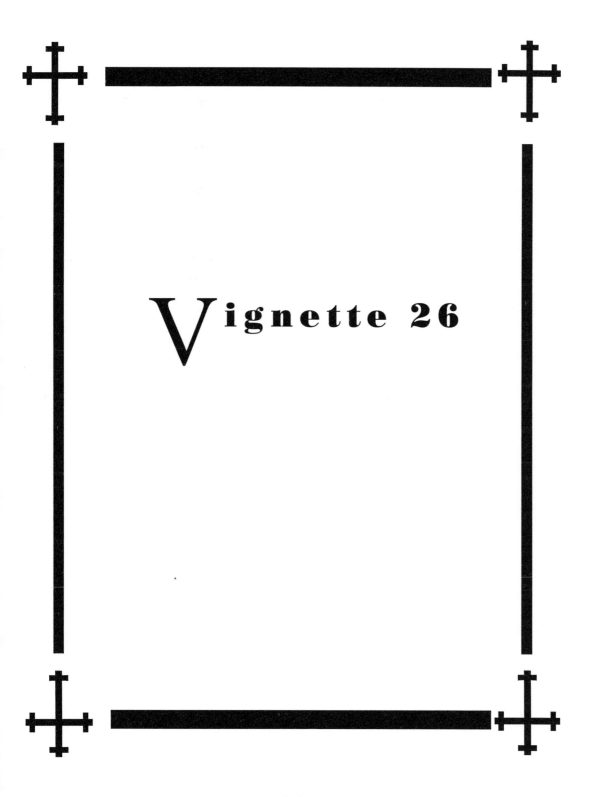

# Vignette 26

# Vignette 26

*You are meeting with a 25-year-old patient and his parents to inform them that he has a diagnosis of schizophrenia. The patient seems disinterested. His mother says that she does not think her son is mentally ill; she thinks that he is just being lazy and is talking rubbish just to get out of doing his share of the domestic chores, and she makes several other critical comments about him. How do you handle the interview and what advice about diagnosis and management do you give?*

265

**You are meeting with a 25-year-old patient and his parents to inform them that he has a diagnosis of schizophrenia. The patient seems disinterested. His mother says that she does not think her son is mentally ill; she thinks that he is just being lazy and is talking rubbish just to get out of doing his share of the domestic chores, and she makes several other critical comments about him. How do you handle the interview and what advice about diagnosis and management do you give?**

1.  Hold the interview in a place where privacy is assured, and carry it out gently, allowing time for the patient and his parents to take in the information and ask questions as they arise.

2.  Give the diagnosis gently:

    - Recall the symptoms and the events that have led up to the diagnosis. Gently challenging the suggestion that these are 'normal' can allow you to state that you think that a disease process is in action and that this is a serious mental illness with a poor outlook.

3.  In talking about the treatment, you need to distinguish what will happen in the short-term from what will happen in the long-term. You will need to give information and discuss the following areas:

    - The nature of the disorder and its natural history
    - Medication
    - Services for patients with schizophrenia and the implications of community care:

        i.   How to obtain help in emergencies/crises

        ii.  Inpatient/day patient and outpatient support

        iii. The various members of the team, e.g. community psychiatric nurses, psychologists

        iv.  Support from social services

        v.   How to obtain longer term help

    - Accommodation
    - Occupation

- Coming to terms with the loss of his bright future
- Coping with stigma
- Help and support for the family.

4. Inform them that there are many other sources of information about the illness, and that the patient and his family can use any that they find helpful:

- Information leaflets from the Royal College of Psychiatrists
- Social work departments
- Self-help groups:

    i. National Schizophrenia Fellowship, MIND, SANE*

Be prepared to take more than one session to cover this, and make it clear to the patient and his parents that you may need to meet on another occasion. If the patient and his parents do not seem to be taking in what you are saying, that may be the time to stop the current interview and delay further discussions until the next meeting.

## Useful addresses

MIND: (National Association for Mental Health)
Granta House, Broadway
London, B15 4BQ
0181-519 2122

NSF: (National Schizophrenia Fellowship)
59a Portabello Road, London W11 3DB
0171-243 3264

SANE (Schizophrenia — A National Emergency)
199 Marylebone Road, London NW1 5QP
0171-724 8000

* SANE = Schizophrenia — A National Emergency

*The patient's mother takes offence and accuses
you of blaming her for causing her son's illness.
She says that she knows that psychiatrists always
blame the mother. How do you respond?*

**The patient's mother takes offence and accuses you of blaming her for causing her son's illness. She says that she knows that psychiatrists always blame the mother. How do you respond?**

1.  Do not take the comment personally:

    ●   Understand that the woman is very upset
    ●   Do not enter into an argument with her.

2.  Sympathetically explain in lay terms, avoiding technical jargon:

    ●   Schizophrenia is currently thought to be a disease process of biological origin, thus it is no-one's 'fault'
    ●   There was previously a theory of a 'schizophrenogenic mother', but this is no longer accepted
    ●   Although the neurodevelopment theory of schizophrenia suggests that obstetric events and other perinatal trauma may be involved in the subsequent development of the disorder, these are clearly not deliberate events.

3.  It is, however, appropriate to explain that:

    ●   Overstimulation can lead to worsening of the positive symptoms
    ●   Understimulation can lead to worsening of the negative symptoms:

        *It is difficult to achieve a balance between these two extremes, nevertheless the stimulation of excessive criticism expressed in an emotional way can aggravate the condition*

    ●   Thus, both parents need to avoid intensely expressed emotion, although it is important to acknowledge that the family will be profoundly distressed by the behaviour of the patient at times, and will need outlets for this distress, such as a friend who is a sympathetic listener, self-help groups, etc.

*The patient's mother expresses the concern that she does not want her boy to become dependent on drugs, especially when no-one knows how they work and the fact that there are horrendous side-effects. How do you deal with her criticisms?*

**The patient's mother expresses the concern that she does not want her boy to become dependent on drugs, especially when no-one knows how they work and the fact that there are horrendous side-effects. How do you deal with her criticisms?**

You reassure her that:

- Neuroleptic drugs are not addictive
- Neuroleptic drugs are a treatment of psychosis, not some indiscriminate 'tranquillisation' to keep him quiet
- Although the exact mechanism of neuroleptic medication is not known, there is plenty of evidence to show that they work as agents which relieve psychosis
- No treatment is without side-effects, and adequate management of the situation involves balancing the risks and benefits of any treatment and reassessing that balance from time to time
- Not everyone suffers side-effects
- The most serious side-effect is Parkinsonism, which can be dealt with.

# Further reading

Creer C, Wing J (1988) *Schizophrenia at Home.* 2nd edn. National Schizophrenia Fellowship, London

Falloon IRH (1992) The psychotherapy of schizophrenia. *Br J Hosp Med* **48**: 164–70

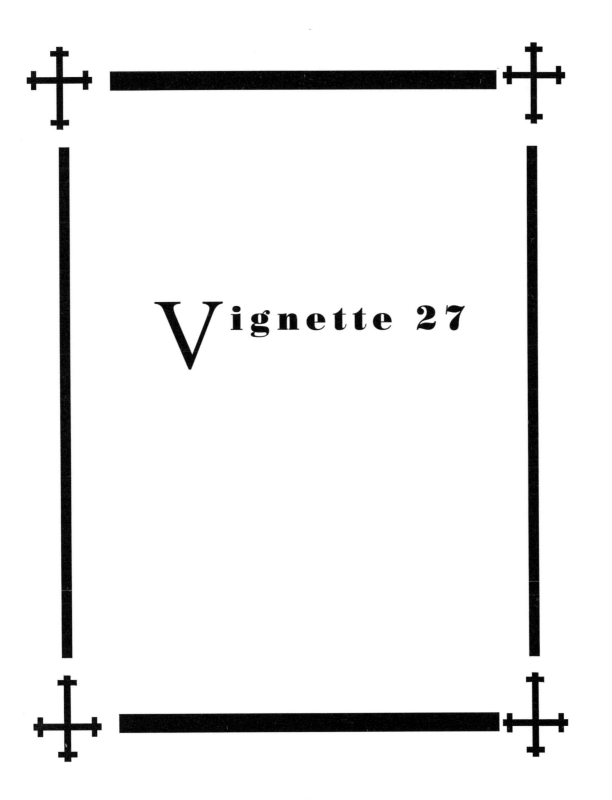

Vignette 27

# Vignette 27

*You are called to the police station at 2 a.m to see a 22-year-old man who has been picked up for interfering with cars. You are told that he has been unable to give a history, as he is rambling and seems disorientated. The police officer has learned from a solicitor that he has used amphetamines and temazepam in the past, but it is not clear when. The patient says that in the past 2 weeks he has taken 'Es (ecstasy; 3,4–methylenediaoxymetamphetamine)' and amitriptyline, both prescribed by a dentist in the high street. On examination, he has dilated pupils, appears perplexed, is talking incoherently and on one occasion seems to see an imaginary cigarette falling on the floor and tries to pick it up. He believes that he is in a hostel for homeless people and that the year is 1976. What might be going on?*

You are called to the police station at 2 a.m to see a 22-year-old man who has been picked up for interfering with cars. You are told that he has been unable to give a history, as he is rambling and seems disorientated. The police officer has learned from a solicitor that he has used amphetamines and temazepam in the past, but it is not clear when. The patient says that in the past 2 weeks he has taken 'Es (ecstasy; 3,4–methylenediaoxymetamphetamine)' and amitriptyline, both prescribed by a dentist in the high street. On examination, he has dilated pupils, appears perplexed, is talking incoherently and on one occasion seems to see an imaginary cigarette falling on the floor and tries to pick it up. He believes that he is in a hostel for homeless people and that the year is 1976. What might be going on?

1.    Drug-induced psychosis:

   ●    Amphetamine, anticholinergic agent, other.

2.    Schizophrenia.

3.    Delirium tremens.

4.    Benzodiazepine withdrawal.

*The police surgeon and approved social worker feel that he should be admitted compulsorily to hospital. You know that the Mental Health Act 1983 does not allow for compulsory admission for the treatment of drug abuse. Do you sign the section form? If so, how do you justify it? If not, how do you manage the situation?*

**The police surgeon and approved social worker feel that he should be admitted compulsorily to hospital. You know that the Mental Health Act 1983 does not allow for compulsory admission for the treatment of drug abuse. Do you sign the section form? If so, how do you justify it? If not, how do you manage the situation?**

In favour of making a medical recommendation for compulsory admission:

- The Mental Health Act 1983 does not allow for treatment of drug dependence, but it does allow for the treatment of mental disorder, which is not further defined:

  > *However, if a patient can be given a diagnosis in accordance with the ICD–10 (World Health Organisation) Classification of Mental and Behavioural Disorders or DSM–IV (American Psychiatric Association), it can be held that the patient is suffering from 'mental disorder' in the terms of the Mental Health Act 1983.*

  > *In these terms, a patient with a diagnosis of drug-induced psychosis or delirium tremens could be construed as falling within the terms of suffering from mental disorder and thus liable to compulsory admission*

- In the situation described, there is not enough information to be certain of the diagnosis, which can only be achieved following further investigations (collateral history, previous notes, urine drug screen), making admission under section 2 for assessment appropriate

- The mental state of the patient is such that he is unable to give or refuse valid consent. Thus compulsory admission is the only option.

Should it be felt that the patient falls outside the terms of the Mental Health Act 1983 (e.g. if he was very well-known, and there was a good history of sharp change in mental state following ingestion of a known illicit psychotropic substance):

- The medical practitioner still has a responsibility for arranging appropriate care for the patient until he is out of medical danger:

    i.    If he was well-known to hostel workers, and they were experienced in looking after the patient in these conditions, he could return there. The doctor would need to that ensure he could be contacted promptly if the situation changes

    ii.   The doctor might admit the patient to hospital (perhaps even a medical ward) if nursing care is needed, assuming that in the absence of the patient's consent he is acting in the interests of the patient, and that should he subsequently be sued, he would claim that he had acted under his duty of care under common law.

## Further reading

The clinical presentation and management of drug-induced psychosis is well covered in standard psychiatric textbooks.

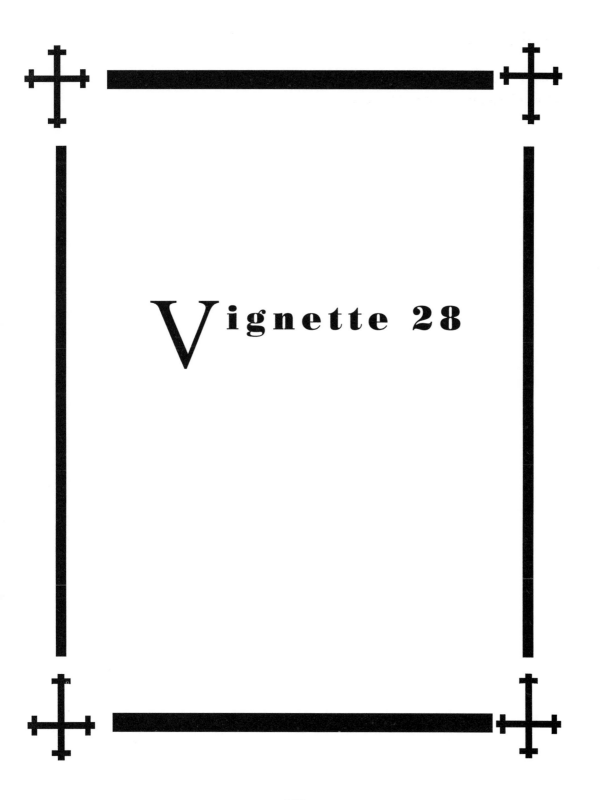

# Vignette 28

# Vignette 28

*You are at a residential home carrying out a domiciliary visit on a patient, when the matron starts talking about another resident, a 72-year-old man who was admitted to the home 4 weeks ago, saying that since he arrived he has been peevish, irritable and unpleasant to look after. What are the diagnostic possibilities?*

You are at a residential home carrying out a domiciliary visit on a patient, when the matron starts talking about another resident, a 72-year-old man who was admitted to the home 4 weeks ago, saying that since he arrived he has been peevish, irritable and unpleasant to look after. What are the diagnostic possibilities?

- Personality clash with staff

- Personality trait

- Adjustment disorder

- Depressive illness

- Acute or chronic brain syndrome.

*You are subsequently called by the GP, who wants to discuss the case with you. After a careful examination of the patient, she says that her provisional diagnosis is that he might be suffering from a depressive illness. She asks you for advice about how depression in the elderly might present. Give examples of different types of presentation of depression in this group.*

You are subsequently called by the GP, who wants to discuss the case with you. After a careful examination of the patient, she says that her provisional diagnosis is that he might be suffering from a depressive illness. She asks you for advice about how depression in the elderly might present. Give examples of different types of presentation of depression in this group.

- Agitated depression

- The importuning dependent person

- The peevish old man

- Psychomotor retardation

- Somatisation/hypochondriasis

- Pseudodementia

- Suicidal behaviour.

*The GP asks if you would assess the patient for her. She offers to be present at the domiciliary visit (DV). How do you assess the patient?*

**The GP asks if you would assess the patient for her. She offers to be present at the domiciliary visit (DV). How do you assess the patient?**

1.     History and mental state examination:

- Your assessment might need to include more attention to physical factors in the aetiology than in a younger person
- Multiple prescribed medication may produce an iatrogenic component to the clinical picture.

1.     Informant history:

- Someone who has known the patient for a long time must be consulted, to confirm that this presentation represents a change from the norm for this person
- The staff of the home may be consulted for observations that might suggest biological features of depression, such as his interpersonal behaviour, although this evidence needs to be weighed carefully as the staff are not dispassionate observers
- The GP may be able to give further medical history, including clues that the change in the mental state might be the result of organic disease (e.g. malignancy) and history of previous mental illness (e.g. previous episodes of depressive illness).

You may have to assess the patient on more than one occasion to determine the diagnosis and institute treatment

*Your diagnosis is that the patient has a depressive illness and you decide to treat him with an antidepressant drug. What aspects of treatment do you need to emphasise, that differ from the treatment of depression in younger patients?*

**Your diagnosis is that the patient has a depressive illness and you decide to treat him with an antidepressant drug. What aspects of treatment do you need to emphasise, that differ from the treatment of depression in younger patients?**

1.  Initially, dosage should be low:

    ● Divided doses of a drug with a long half-life might be more appropriate than a single, daily dose (e.g. giving amitriptyline 75 mg twice daily rather than 159 mg at night, to reduce the risk of higher peak plasma levels that could lead to falls in the middle of the night).

2.  There should be careful observation for side-effects, which are more prominent in the elderly:

    ● Tricyclic side-effects:

        i.   Postural hypotension, urinary retention, constipation, precipitation of glaucoma and precipitation of confusional state all occur frequently

    ● Serotonergic side-effects:

        i.   Some clinicians have observed a serotonergic syndrome following administration of a selective serotonin reuptake inhibitor, although this appears to be infrequent.

3.  You should be prepared for the possibility of a longer time before the patient responds to the drug (although many patients respond as quickly as younger people).

4.  Emotional support may be enlisted from the staff of the home:

    ● Older people do adapt to new situations, although the period of time might be longer
    ● In-depth dynamic psychotherapy plays a less useful part in this patient group
    ● The staff of the home may be willing to supervise or even dispense medication.

5.  Advice and explanation to the staff about the diagnosis and the disorder will often facilitate their caring for the patient in a more sympathetic manner.

# Further reading

Benbow SM (1992) Management of depression in the elderly. *Br J Hosp Med* **48**: 726–31

Burns A, Baldwin R (1994) Prescribing psychotropic drugs for the elderly. *Adv Psych Treat* **1**: 23–31

Collins E, Katona C, Orrell M (1994) Diagnosis and management of depression in old age. *Focus on Depression* **2**: 1–5

Howard R (1993) Depression or dementia? *Focus on Depression* **1**: 1–3

Jacoby R, Oppenheimer C eds (1991) *Psychiatry in the Elderly*. Oxford University Press, Oxford

Old Age Depression Interest Group (1993) How long should the elderly take antidepressants? A double-blind, placebo-controlled study of continuation/prophylaxis therapy. *Br J Psychiatry* **162**: 175–82

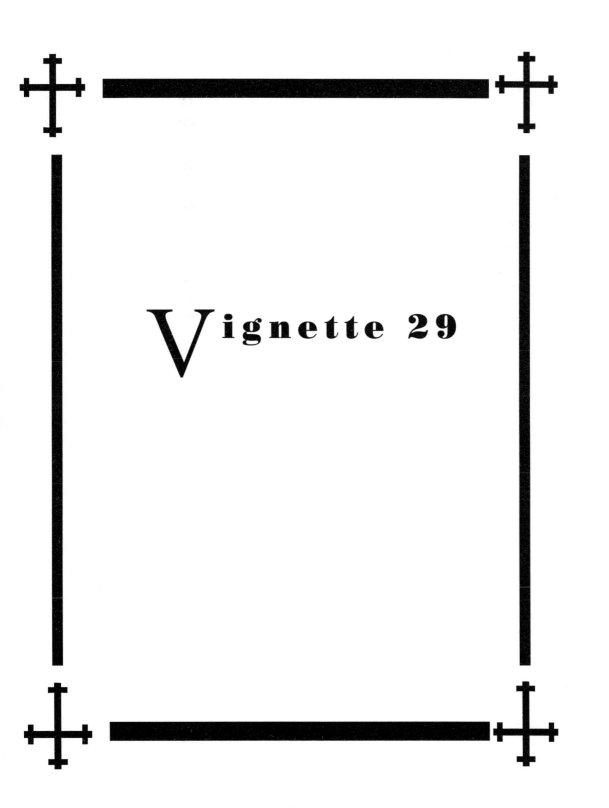

# Vignette 29

# Vignette 29

*You are providing a consultation service to a local general practice in their surgery when one of the GPs asks your advice about a 31-year-old married woman with two young children. She has metastases from a breast carcinoma, is cachectic with back pain, controlled by non-steroidal anti-inflammatory agents, and has poor appetite. The GP says that the last time he saw the patient he wondered if she was becoming depressed and asks you what features might suggest that depressive illness is supervening on her malignant disease. How do you reply?*

You are providing a consultation service to a local general practice in their surgery when one of the GPs asks your advice about a 31-year-old married woman with two young children. She has metastases from a breast carcinoma, is cachectic with back pain, controlled by non-steroidal anti-inflammatory agents, and has poor appetite. The GP says that the last time he saw the patient he wondered if she was becoming depressed and asks you what features might suggest that depressive illness is supervening on her malignant disease. How do you reply?

Elements that typify depressive disorder

1.  Anxiety and depressive symptoms:

    - If becoming more intense
    - If the patient conveys a sense that anxiety and depressive symptoms are out of proportion to what is happening
    - If accompanied by regressive behaviour not normal for the patient
    - Patient seems to be more or unusually dependent
    - While anorexia, weight loss and lethargy are more likely to be the result of the cancer process, psychosexual disorders and sleep disorder (except as a result of inadequately controlled pain) are less likely to be so.

2.  Psychosis:

    - Hallucinations, delusions.

Ensure that organic brain disorder is non coexistent (more suggestive of brain metastases than depressive illness).

*What aspects of the management of this patient need particular attention?*

## What aspects of the management of this patient need particular attention?

1. Nutrition as adequate as possible:

   - May need food supplements (e.g. ®Ensure)
   - Better nutrition will make pain more tolerable and mood less low.

2. Adequate pain relief.

3. Use of an antidepressant drug:

   - If supervening depressive illness
   - As an adjunct to difficulty in keeping pain control (e.g. if addition of an opiate leaves her excessively drowsy at doses required for adequate analgesia).

1. Support for her and her family:

   - The GP
   - District nurse
   - Macmillan nurse
   - Social worker (also for financial advice and childcare issues)
   - Self-help groups
   - Pastoral if belonging to a church or other religious organisation
   - Friends , who might provide personal support and help with practical tasks.

5. Adequate information about what is happening to her, and what her options are.

# Further reading

Brugha TS (1993) Depression in the terminally ill. *Br J Hosp Med* **50**: 175–81

Greer S (1985) Cancer: psychiatric aspects. In: Granville-Grossman K, ed. *Recent Advances in Clinical Psychiatry*. 5. Churchill Livingstone, London

Greer S, Moorey S, Baruch JDR *et al* (1992) Adjuvant psychological therapy for patients with cancer: a prospective randomised trial. *Br Med J* **304**: 675–80

Harrison J, Maguire P (1994) Predictors of psychiatric morbidity in cancer patients. *Br J Psychiatry* **165**: 593–8

Maguire P (1980) Effect of counselling on the psychiatric morbidity associated with mastectomy. *Br Med J* **ii**: 1454

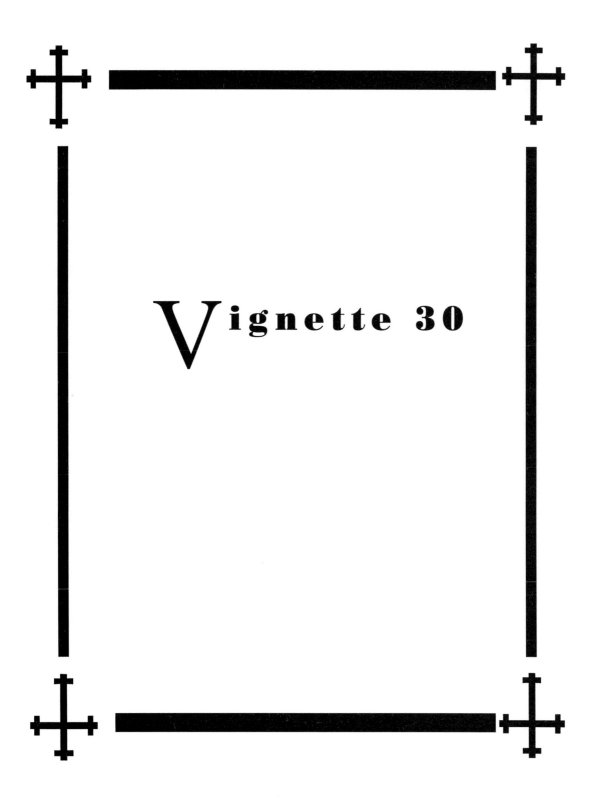

# Vignette 30

# Vignette 30

*You are sitting in a multidisciplinary team meeting when one of the community psychiatric nurses raises her concern about one of her patients. The patient is a 42-year-old woman with a 15-year history of depressive episodes who has been managed in the community. She complains of constant strong feelings of depressed mood, with poor sleep, slightly low appetite (without weight loss) and mild constipation. She seems to take no pleasure in anything, although she does manage to watch `soap operas' on the television regularly, and is able to keep her house `spic and span' for her overbearing and unsympathetic husband, who expects his dinner on the table when he gets in. Her two teenage sons seem to treat the home as a hotel, and she feels that they do not appreciate her. The nurse is concerned that the patient has complained that her depression was becoming more intense. The patient has mentioned the return of suicidal feelings, which she has had on and off for periods of months during the time of her illness, and which she has occasionally given in to by taking overdoses, with one serious occasion 4 years ago. What aspects do you need to consider in the management of this patient?*

You are sitting in a multidisciplinary team meeting when one of the community psychiatric nurses raises her concern about one of her patients. The patient is a 42-year-old woman with a 15-year history of depressive episodes who has been managed in the community. She complains of constant strong feelings of depressed mood, with poor sleep, slightly low appetite (without weight loss) and mild constipation. She seems to take no pleasure in anything, although she does manage to watch 'soap operas' on the television regularly, and is able to keep her house 'spic and span' for her overbearing and unsympathetic husband, who expects his dinner on the table when he gets in. Her two teenage sons seem to treat the home as a hotel, and she feels that they do not appreciate her. The nurse is concerned that the patient has complained that her depression was becoming more intense. The patient has mentioned the return of suicidal feelings, which she has had on and off for periods of months during the time of her illness, and which she has occasionally given in to by taking overdoses, with one serious occasion 4 years ago. What aspects do you need to consider in the management of this patient?

1. Support to avoid the patient acting on suicidal impulses and relief from environmental stresses:

   - Hospital admission, either as an inpatient or a day patient, or frequent outpatient follow-up:

     i. To provide additional counselling, both formal and informal

     ii. To provide the opportunity for the expression of feelings about current stresses and long-term difficulties, both verbally (e.g. day hospital groups) and non-verbally (e.g. art therapy)

   - Help in increasing other supports (assistance of spouse or close friend, awareness and use of self-help groups or the Samaritans).

2. Dynamic psychotherapy, if the patient can tolerate it:

   - Individual psychotherapy
   - Group psychotherapy.

3.    Supportive psychotherapy:

- Cognitive–behavioural therapy
- Assertiveness skills
- Marital or family therapy:

    i.    Either as formal therapy or as exploratory meetings

- Systematic desensitisation
- Relaxation techniques.

4.    Psychopharmacology:

- Antidepressant medication as prime therapy:

    i.    Tricyclic antidepressant drugs (TCAs), monoamine oxidase inhibitors (MAOIs) including reversible inhibitors of monoamine (RIMAs), and selective serotonin reuptake inhibitors (SSRIs)

- Anxiolytic therapy:

    i.    Low-dose neuroleptic medication may be helpful, although with an increased risk of tardive dyskinesia; alternatively, administer a benzodiazepine, although in this patient it would be important to watch for the risk of addiction.

*The multidisciplinary team contains a wide range of professionals, although there is a feeling that, as the doctor in the group, you are the team leader. What are the principles of team leadership in such a group?*

**The multidisciplinary team contains a wide range of professionals, although there is a feeling that, as the doctor in the group, you are the team leader. What are the principles of team leadership in such a group?**

1. Encourage all members to attend regularly and on time:

   - This shows that the group is taking its responsibility to perform the agreed task seriously(e.g. review of the clinical state of patients in its care).

2. Assist in ensuring mutual respect for all members of the team:

   - Encourage each individual to speak freely, and protect anyone who seems to feel insecure and is apparently being 'got at' by another member of the team
   - Welcome new members and visitors
   - Encourage democratic decisions where possible (e.g. the team should be asked to decide collectively whether a proposed visitor, such as a member of another health-care team, may sit in on a team meeting on a certain day).

3. Assist in clarifying roles:

   - Distinguish between the role of the keyworker and the role of specialist:

     i. The **key worker** is the team member who takes responsibility for assessing the patient, ensuring that the patient receives the treatment offered by the team, being a first point of call for the patient as problems arise and evaluating progress. This task can be performed by any member of the team, and is not specific to any particular function

     ii. The **specialist function** arises when one member of the team has a specific skill to offer that other members of the team cannot offer. It is complicated, as there are situations when team members from more than one discipline can offer specialist help, e.g. psychiatrists, psychiatric nurses, psychologists and social workers do take courses to become proficient in cognitive therapy

- Be clear about your own specialist functions as a psychiatrist. These should include:

  i. The ability to carry out a comprehensive assessment taking into account biological, social and psychological factors

  ii. Ability to offer advice about general medical problems

  iii. Ability to offer advice about psychopharmacology

  iv. Acting as a repository of the psychiatric and scientific literature

  v. A willingness to adopt the function of team leader

  vi. Legal responsibility for the care of the patient.

4. Chair team meetings:

- Clarify the rules of the meeting, e.g. when it will start and finish, what the agenda will be, whether there will be a coffee break
- Ensure that each member of the team has the opportunity to speak
- Ensure, as far as possible, that each person has the same amount of time to speak if he/she wants to
- Be prepared to interrupt to keep to the allocated time
- Be prepared to interrupt any speaker or argument that is veering away from the task in hand
- Ensure that the meeting overall keeps to time — this can be made easier by setting the agenda clearly at the start and the time to discuss each patient, prioritising if necessary.

*One of the longstanding members of the team is a social worker who does not believe that drugs should be prescribed to treat an oppressed woman in what is, on the surface at least, a dysfunctional family in which the woman is being labelled as mentally ill to scapegoat the systemic dysfunction. Furthermore, this woman has already taken antidepressant medication for long periods without any apparent improvement, and the social worker cannot see the point in giving her any more drugs. How do you explain the rationale for further prescribing of antidepressant medication, and what scientific evidence is there to support this as being appropriate for this patient?*

One of the longstanding members of the team is a social worker who does not believe that drugs should be prescribed to treat an oppressed woman in what is, on the surface at least, a dysfunctional family in which the woman is being labelled as mentally ill to scapegoat the systemic dysfunction. Furthermore, this woman has already taken antidepressant medication for long periods without any apparent improvement, and the social worker cannot see the point in giving her any more drugs. How do you explain the rationale for further prescribing of antidepressant medication, and what scientific evidence is there to support this as being appropriate for this patient?

Explain tactfully that you are advising the administration of antidepressant medication because there is scientific evidence that it will help the patient, and not because you are under the impression that all problems in the world can be solved by pills.

- There is evidence that antidepressant drugs help patients who have syndromes of depression as defined in psychiatric classifications, such as ICD–10 (World Health Organisation) and DSM–IV (American Psychiatric Association)

    i.    For example, the Medical Research Council trial of the treatment of acute depression showed that treatment with imipramine or electroconvulsive therapy was more effective than placebo (Medical Research Council, 1965)

- There is evidence in the case of all the drugs that are licensed for the treatment of depressive illness that they have efficacy at least as good as the standard tricyclic antidepressant drugs (imipramine and amitriptyline are usually taken as examples of standard treatment):

    i.    There are numerous examples of such studies and you should know a few: drug company representatives will be only too happy to offer an example in support of their own drug

- There is evidence that antidepressant medication can help even when the depression seems to have a psychosocial precipitant and maintaining factors

- More recent evidence suggests that patients with chronic depression fare better in a modest way if they take antidepressant medication rather than if this is not prescribed (see Montgomery, 1994).

NB: An arrogant approach to this type of question might lead an examiner to question your suitability to be accepted as a Member of the Royal College of Psychiatrists.


# Further reading

## Antidepressant medication

Medical Research Council (1965) Clinical trial of the treatment of depressive illness. Report to the Medical Research Council by its Clinical Psychiatry Committee. *Br Med J* i: 881–6

Mindham RHS, Howland C, Shepherd M (1973) An evaluation of continuation therapy with tricyclic antidepressants in depressive illness. *Psychol Med* **3**: 5–17

Montgomery SA (1994) Long-term treatment of depression. *Br J Psychiatry* **165** (suppl. 26): 31–6

## Management

Bhugra D, Burns A, eds (1992) *Management Training for Psychiatrists*. Gaskell, London

Salmon G (1994) Working in a multidisciplinary team: need it be so difficult? (personal view) *Br Med J* **309**: 1520

Simpson J (1994) Doctors and management — why bother? *Br Med J* **309**: 1505–8

# Bibliography and Further Reading

## Books containing patient management problem examples

Fottrell E (1983) *Case Histories in Psychiatry*. Churchill Livingstone, London

Green B ed. (1993) *The MRCPsych Study Manual*. Kluwer Academic, Lancaster

Johnson BA (1991) *Solving Conundrums in Clinical Psychiatry*. Kluwer Academic, Lancaster

Levi MI (1992) *PMPs for the MRCPsych Part II*. Kluwer Academic, Lancaster


## MRCPsych Examination Related

Many pieces are contained in the regular MRCPsych supplements of the British Journal of Hospital Medicine


## General Psychiatric Background

American Psychiatric Association (1994) Diagnostic and Statistical Manual of Mental Disorders — 4 edn. (DSM—IV). American Psychiatric Association, Washington USA

Cookson J, Crammer J, Heine B (1993) The Use of Drugs in Psychiatry. Gaskell, London

Gelder M, Gath D, Mayou R (1989) Oxford Textbook of Psychiatry. Oxford Medical Publications, Oxford

Henderson AS (1988) An Introduction to Social Psychiatry. Oxford Medical Publications, Oxford

Lishman WA (1987) Organic Psychiatry — The Psychological Consequences of Cerebral Disorder. Blackwell Scientific Publications, Oxford

WHO (1992) The ICD—10 Classification of Mental and Behavioural Disorders. Clinical Descriptions and Diagnostic Guidelines. World Health Organization, Geneva

# List of Vignettes